The Pornographer

Restif de la Bretonne

Translated By Richard Robinson

Sunny Lou Publishing Company
Portland, Oregon, USA
http://www.sunnyloupublishing.com

2nd Edition: March 28, 2024
Original Publication Date: July 19, 2021

ISBN: 978-1-955392-64-8

* * *

This translation from French is based on
the Gosse Junior, & Pinet, Librairies de S.A.S. publication
of *Le Pornographe,* La Haie, 1770.

Contents

Foreword

Sed ut perspiciatis, unde omnis iste natus error sit voluptatem accusantium doloremque laudantium, totam rem aperiam eaque ipsa, quae ab illo inventore veritatis et quasi architecto beatae vitae dicta sunt, explicabo. Nemo enim ipsam voluptatem, quia voluptas sit, aspernatur aut odit aut fugit, sed quia consequuntur magni dolores eos, qui ratione voluptatem sequi nesciunt, neque porro quisquam est, qui dolorem ipsum, quia dolor sit, amet, consectetur, adipisci velit, sed quia non numquam eius modi tempora incidunt, ut labore et dolore magnam aliquam quaerat voluptatem. Ut enim ad minima veniam, quis nostrum exercitationemullam corporis suscipit laboriosam, nisi ut aliquid ex ea commodi consequatur? Quis autem vel eum iure reprehenderit, qui in ea voluptate velit esse, quam nihil molestiae consequatur, vel illum, qui dolorem eum fugiat, quo voluptas nulla pariatur? [33] At vero eos et accusamus et iusto odio dignissimos ducimus, qui blanditiis praesentium voluptatum deleniti atque corrupti, quos dolores et quas molestias excepturi sint, obcaecati cupiditate non provident, similique sunt in culpa, qui officia deserunt mollitia animi, id est laborum et dolorum fuga. Et harum quidem rerum facilis est et expedita distinctio. Nam libero tempore, cum soluta nobis est eligendi optio, cumque nihil impedit, quo minus id, quod maxime placeat, facere possimus, omnis voluptas assumenda est, omnis dolor repellendus. Temporibus autem quibusdam et aut officiis debitis aut rerum necessitatibus saepe eveniet, ut et voluptates repudiandae sint ct molestiae non recusandae. Itaque earum rerum hic tenetur a sapiente delectus, ut aut reiciendis voluptatibus maiores alias consequatur aut perferendis doloribus asperiores repellat.

    – Cicero, 45 BC (*de Finibus Bonorum et Malorum*)

The Pornographer

or **An Honest Man's Ideas on a Plan of Rules for Prostitutes**

Suitable for Preventing the Misfortunes that the Prostitution of Women Occasions: with Historical Notes and Justifications

"Take the Least Evil for a Good."
– Machiavelli, The Prince, Chapter XXI.

Original Publisher's Preface

The idea of this Work was not born in a French head: there is reason to presume that an English manuscript, which several people from London had seen, is the type on which it is modeled. The first Author was named Lewis Moore: here is his history.

An Englishman, young, opulent, fit and trim, wanted to see the world and educate himself at the school of all Nations of Europe: he came to Paris. That city appeared to him much better than it was renowned to be; everything convinced him that the Paradise that Mohammed promised for his elect is nothing in comparison to the French Capital for a man who can distribute gold with both hands. For five years, he could not resolve to end that enchanting sojourn. But his revenue, although considerable, was well inferior to his expenses: fantasies about a principal Mistress absorbed three quarters of them. He saw himself finally in the necessity of making a change; he started with that capricious woman; then he forced himself to fill the void that that sacrifice left in his heart, with facile, varied pleasures, and which cost less. Shameful maladies overpowered him. Completely spent at thirty years old, he returned to his Fatherland, to bemoan his errors: it was then that he undertook to trace out a Plan of reform, which he could not profit by. He put at the head of his plan the following advice:

"I was a libertine; I am no longer. Barely in the middle of my career, I glimpsed the end. Very short pleasures were followed by long and cruel maladies. I had recourse to antidotes, to that powerful mineral, which bears the name of the Planet closest to the Sun, to Charlatans; alas! in vain. No longer seeing anything to do for myself, I resolved to be useful for others, by making my ideas public, on the means to diminish the inconveniences of a certain condition that revolts nature, but which I feel is impossible to destroy. Would that one could, by a useful Establishment, grab hold of the evil at its source, and protect our young Citizens in an efficacious manner from a destructive venom that is sure to bring me to an early death! I hereby declare that I leave the half of my property for contributing to it, if ever one resolves on realizing my ideas."

– Lewis Moore

(His Plan then followed, almost entirely like that of the French: it terminated like this:)

"If it is sometimes permitted to a simple Citizen to propose his ideas for the general good, it is without a doubt that, when he does it, he does it with all the respect due to the Government under which he lives, and when he has cause to fear that the abuses whose reformation he desires tend to deprive him of his sweetest hope *of having healthy, robust, and virtuous children.*"

Such is also my goal, in giving this Version of a similar Plan that its Author was going to bury forever in obscurity. Honest fellows, looking on my endeavor like an effect of my zeal and of my love for humanity, will do nothing but render me justice.

The work, composed of eleven Letters, is divided into five parts or sections. In the first, one avows the necessity of tolerating Prostitutes in the Capital and other large cities of the Realm. The second contains a detail of the inseparable inconveniences of Prostitution, even while following the outlined Plan. One discusses then those that accompany it today, and the Reader will agree that they are frightening.

One proposes the remedy in the third section, which contains the Rules. One will see there that a House of Prostitution, well administered, which would collect all those miserable souls, the scandal of Society, could be self-sufficient; to diminish the abuse that the wisdom of the laws tolerate, without causing any of the inconveniences that a reform of another kind would occasion; and to contribute to the re-establishment of public decency and integrity, from which it seems public mores are insensibly removed.

The fourth section addresses Objections; clarifies, presents some Articles.

In the fifth, one recapitulates the Receipts and Expenses.

It is by those five sections that one proves the proposition that the Establishment, beyond the advantage that men derive from it in order to conserve their health, their property, and even their mores, can also be useful in another manner.

In the course of this work, one has placed some unimportant notes; others much more important are found, that have been placed at the end; they will form a second part. The Readers will find some historical traits on the mores of the Ancients; the origin and state of Prostitution among early peoples; its current state; examples of revolting abuses among us; the manner in which public women were governed in the Middle Ages; one will be convinced that those vile and miserable creatures were not always abandoned like today... But is it possible that the worthy and vigilant Magistracy, which governs the Capital of France, should take the trouble to delve into the minute and disgusting details requiring too considerable a number of Debauchees?

Singular Ideas

The Pornographer (or
Prostitution Reformed)

Part One

Fragment of a Letter

From Madame Des Tianges to her husband.

Paris, April 6, 176*.

… Yes, I am very content; my *pupil* stands up to the test marvelously. Honor takes the ascendent in his soul, over the habit of vice. He was telling me yesterday, that he found me charming, but that his attachment to Monsieur *Des Tianges* prevented him from seeing in the wife of so respectable and so true a friend, anything but a cherished sister. Let's keep our fingers crossed, my dear friend, for a heart that doubtless was never made to go astray. The regrettable consequences that his original disorders produced will have disgusted him. His conversation most often turns to the reform he would desire to see instilled in public mores on that score. When he runs into one of those vile creatures... he shudders; then his face blushes. All that he needs now is an honest, legitimate love, to succeed in affirming him in goodness. Since I believe that I can do it without imprudence, I will lead him to Ursule's convent. My sister is as dear to you as to me; her joy will augment our own, and I am sure that D'Alzan will make her happy, if he wants to...

I will be, my dear friend, all my glorious life bearing the title of your wife, happy thereby to be your lover.

– Adelaïde

Second Letter

From D'Alzan to Des Tianges.

Paris, April 10, 176*.

You do know, my dear Des Tianges, that your absence is too long, don't you? What! Newly married to the loveliest, most seductive of women, you are not afraid of three long months! In all honesty, my dear friend, I find that if it is not for having too much confidence in the virtue of your charming wife, it is at least for having too much in your own merit. In the century that we live in... but think on it! in our days Penelope would not have lasted one week, and Lucretia would have been merely a coquette: lovers always at the table, always drunk, quite seductive objects! the coarse *Sextus* menaces her verbally, a poignard in hand... my faith! that fierce attempt today would find a *Lucretia* in a girl of the *Opera*. Our polite mores are much more fatal to a husband's honor: we have shaken off the yoke of prejudices: conjugal fidelity was already no longer one of our grandmothers' virtues, and now! one marries as one pays a New Year's compliment, for that is the custom; but fundamentally, one hardly cares for one another as before. Nothing is easier; it must be confessed though that society has taken a tone for the better: in half a century... the extraordinary things one will be able to see in half a century!... You did not get married like that, the beautiful Adelaïde and you: you got married for the best of reasons: I bewail it in all honesty. A young wife, more fetching than the Graces, vivacious, cheerful, made for the world and made for love, lives in retreat because her husband is absent, desires his return imbecilely, counts the weeks, the days, the hours, that must pass without seeing him, while she could... yes, while she could imitate others instead, forgive me for saying so. I would not try to persuade her; I believe she is incorrigible. But if I wanted to, what fine things I could tell her! First of all, I would site the Greeks, I would tell her emphatically: the Lacedaemonians,[1] that proud and courageous people, the honor and example of the human species, thought as at present, and the women of Sparta were... common to everyone. I would prove it to her with a copy of *Plutarch* in hand. From there, I would come to the polite century of Augustus; I would have her see Livia, going, although pregnant, from the arms of her husband, into the bed of the happy Roman tyrant: I would show her the Romans, those conquerors of the world, making a game of divorce and adultery: their women flying intrepidly over *the fourteen rows of seats in the Orchestra*,[2] to go pick up a rascal from among the dregs of the people. Agrippina, Julia, forgetting the status of mothers... But there's too much of that, and the raillery goes further than I care to take it. Your dear Adelaïde would not see in those too infamous examples but degraded humanity, indignantly demeaned under the dirty feet of proud impudence.

---

[1]Lacedaemonians: or Spartans particularly.

[2]Original footnote: *Domina... usque ab orchestrâ quatuordecim transilit, & in extremâ plebe quæri quod diligat... Ego adhuc servo numquam succubui... Viderint matronæ quæ flagellorum vestigia osculantur; ego etiam, si ancilla sum, umquam tamen, nisi inequestribus sedeo... Ne hoc dii sinant, ut amplexus meos in crucem mittam!* – Petronius

See how over the course of time men have substituted an unjust, unbridled license for a generous freedom. There are some centuries however in which vices are more veiled, because one still blushes for them: others in which one scandalously lifts the mask. Whereupon we arrive at today, – are our mores more openly similar to that excess of indecency that they were seen to be at, at the fall of the Roman Republic?

Without repeating for the thousandth time that the more men gather together in large numbers, the more their fortunes become unequal, and by necessary consequence the softer, more effeminate, and more dissolute some people become; while others become base, servile, and easy to corrupt; I see in it a direct cause of something: *Prostitution*, such as it is tolerated among us.

I will develop my thought for you at greater length: but come back to Paris, and we will chat. I will employ the rest of my paper to speak to you about your dear, respectable wife.

We are almost always together, as you encouraged us to be; and the lesson I have drawn from our frequent conversations is that I am still convinced that there are women worthy of being adored, I who did not believe that there were any truly estimable ones. Unjust preventative that I blush at, and that I wish to expiate by making a choice like yours. Madame Des Tianges did not convert me by syllogisms, logical reasonings; but by her conduct: she opened her heart to me: O heaven! what a treasure of innocence, tenderness, and generosity! Your happiness has excited my desires; but I do not envy you for it, my friend, you deserve it too much. And then, to tell you the truth, unreservedly, I have just learnt that your wife has a sister, as lovely as she is: that clarified some certain comments that Madame Des Tianges made to me, which I did not understand. Tomorrow we are going to visit the convent of that pretty Recluse: I will see her: the impatience I have to see her surprises me; I take that for a good sign: it is she clearly who must make me feel that felicity, which I had no conception of before your virtuous wife had received me. Hurry up and come back, my good friend; I will have need of someone to put in a good word for me. Would that I might someday join, to the name of friend that you honor me with, the title of brother! I am yours entirely, my dear friend.

— D'ALZAN

Third Letter

From the same.

April 20.

Is everything going okay, given you have not come back yet? Ah! my friend, can one live separated for so long from what one loves? Love and friendship demand equally their violated rights. *Business*! you have *business*, you say? Eh, well, let it follow its course, and return to your wife, and friend, who are in need of you. The dignity with which you speak *of that business* that keeps you, and in which province even? in *Poitou*! does it not seem to you that it is a matter of your money or your life?...

I have seen the charming Ursule. Ah! Des Tianges, I would have accused you of an injustice for having kept hidden from me so rare a treasure, if my conscience had not cried out that I was unworthy of her. My good friend, what pleasure I had on meeting her! As soon as we arrived, the tower opened, Ursule came out, and the two charming sisters flew into each other's arms; they caressed each other for a long time like tender doves. Then your kind companion presented me to her sister as your friend and hers. I was beside myself: the confusion that I could not prevent told me that I had just found my vanquisher, and that the fairer sex was going to be avenged. I wanted to pay her a compliment: I lacked all common sense. Madame Des Tianges laughed with all her heart; and you know how pretty she is when she laughs; Ursule blushed; and her disconcerted friend kept quiet. I gathered my wits however after a moment, and as soon as I thought I could speak my heart, without trying to be clever, I expressed myself in a way that gave honor to the two of them: at least that is what your incomparable wife obligingly told me. What am I saying, *incomparable*! Oh, the word is no longer used today: I would have said it yesterday still without scruple; but today... My friend, Ursule resembles her too much not to equal her... She speaks of you, that charming Ursule, with such praise!... I am sure she will defer to all your advice. Come back then, my dear friend, come back, in order to dispose her in my favor... However, I would have some remorse. For her little sister just informed me that your business in Poitiers is so worthy of a heart like yours; so that, in truth, I have some misgivings about wanting to deprive those orphans, whose affairs you are managing, whose rights you defend, of your support. You see; I am beginning to walk in your footsteps. That is the first effect of the feelings that the darling Ursule's charms have inspired in me.

Nevertheless, wrapped up in your virtue, you grow tired, and I am sure that you would desire us all by your side. We would desire it as well. But given the duties that your wife fulfills here with respect to your parents, the thing becomes impossible; I will try to get an upper hand on my natural laziness and to respond to the invitation you made me to treat of the moral point that I had touched on in my last letter.

I said to you, if I remember correctly, that our mores could become indecent, and that they are very corrupt: I advanced that the manner in which public women and kept women live in the capital and in our large cities, mixing amongst us, was a direct cause. Given that I write to you to help you take your mind off yourself, I will not make a Dissertation: but I will try to put some order to my PORNOGNOMONY,[3] as much as is needed to be understood...

I see you smiling: the half-barbarous word PORNOGRAPHER[4] traces itself on your lips. Go on, my dear friend, smile – I'm not afraid. Why should it be shameful to speak about abuses that one undertakes to reform?

PORNOGNOMONY

As you know, my dear friend; there is a cruel malady, brought to Europe from the island of *Haiti*[5] by *Christopher Columbus,* and it is perpetuated among

---

[3]Original footnote: This Greek word means *Rules of Conduct for Places of Debauchery.*

[4]Original footnote: That is to say, a "Writer who treats of prostitution."

[5]Original footnote: Haiti, at present Santo Domingo, one of the Antilles, where the *big sister of small pox* [scil. syphilis] is endemic, and as if natural, because of the quality of the aliments, the heat of the climate, or the incontinence of its ancient inhabitants. It is in this way that the other scourge, named *small pox,* is proper to Arabia: it resulted from the conquests of Mohammed; the *Crusaders* brought it to Europe on return from the *Holy Land:* and such are the fruits that the human race has acquired from the *Crusades* and the discovery of the *New World.*

those miserable wretches whom the continual approach of Foreigners makes as if almost necessary in large cities.[6] It is in this way that nature, the common mother of all men, seemed, from the first instant of an unjust usurpation, to want to avenge the rights of her children, on the barbarous men who fleeced their own brothers of a sacred patrimony. A punishment that is as just as it is terrible, and that ought to make us regard those so-called heroes, for whom our hemisphere was not enough, as the scourges of the human race. The ancients were no less ambitious than we were; but they were much wiser: they had been cast by rough weather onto the different shores of America; they made however no use of that discovery. Eh! Who knows the real reason for that frightening maxim that they established subsequently, that nobody could cross the Torrid Zone without dying? Their experience, less fatal than ours, had doubtless instructed them: those who had been infected with *venereal disease*, either on the islands or on the continent of the New World, perished without communicating it; because they had the good faith to make their horrible ravages known in time. But if it were a prejudice, that terror that the Ancients had, it was a happy one: would that it had pleased God in these latter days to have stopped the first madman who dared cross the seas!

Given that the damage is done, it is merely a

---

[6]The introduction of syphilis into Europe is commonly dated at some time after the discovery of the New World by Christopher Columbus, in 1492. This is not to say that Europe did not have, prior to then, other sexually transmittable infections. See *Note L* for instance.

question now of finding the cure. Of the two means that present themselves, that of *separation from society*, as was previously done with *lepers,*[7] *all those whom the contagion had attacked*, it was practicable only at the time of arrival of the virus in Europe from Haiti; the *second* which would consist *in collecting in one place, where one could answer for them, all* PUBLIC WOMEN, is less difficult to effect; it is more efficacious, more important, as it would strike at the ill at its source. A Rule for Prostitutes, which would procure their sequestration, without abolishing them, without putting them out of reach of all the estates, at the same time keeping them in business, perhaps a little too agreeable, but certain, and less outrageous to nature. Such a Rule, I say, would have, insofar as I think, an inevitable effect on the extirpation of the *virus*; and would produce perhaps even other advantages, that one does not expect by any measure. To give birth to a good from the last degree of corruption in public mores would be a masterwork of human wisdom, an imitation of Divinity.

The upright man, a citizen of big cities, regards with regret the reigning there of an abuse of the most sacred pleasures; of those pleasures destined to repair the losses that humankind suffers daily. That abuse, always tolerated, although its appalling ravages robs the state of so many subjects, is a stumbling block, where the wisdom of our laws breaks down. All the effort and all the prudence of a wise father cannot keep from peril a son whose peers lead him astray, and whom their misfortune even instructs him

---

[7]Original scholium: See the *Note A* at the end.

only in part, if he does not share it. An overexuberant youth, as you know, my dear friend, seeks pleasure, and meets only sorrow, or often death. From the farthest reaches of their provinces, young men run to the capital, attracted by ambition, or led by duty; and those souls, novices yet, find themselves, in the middle of a large world, at the center of polite society, more exposed to danger than among barbarians or wild beasts.

In fact, how can they resist? A shapely girl sets them on edge; a charming smile lights up her deceptive little face: her breast, merely suggestive, tempts as much as her mouth and hand: she has a svelte and thin waist. With art, she lets one catch a glimpse of her fine leg, and her little foot which a cute mule half covers. However, those seductive attractions are practically nothing compared to those other things of hers that a loathsome old woman talks up. She approaches them stealthily; she speaks to them, she detains them: honey is on her lips, poison is in her words, contagion is exhaled from her impure soul. If they allow themselves to listen to her, they are done for. She has girls at her place whose enchanting faces instill confusion and burning desires into every heart. The only thing that will embarrass you is the choice: there are all the nuances of youth; flanks that in the age of innocence have already acquired all the talents of the miserable souls they have been given over to. Like those young Slaves whom the Georgian or Circassian Tartary inhabitant raises for seraglios in Persia or Turkey, and whom he instructs from infancy to caress the master who ought to buy them, they have on their lips all the words of debauchery; they have lubricious attitudes, without understanding a thing about it. Those charms, which Nature has made the sweet apanage of their sex, are not even fully developed and already a burning desire is happy to exploit[8] them: innocent and unfortunate creatures who are destined to re-kindle in old libertines, more worn-out and corrupted than ugly, a languishing voluptuousness, spent sensations. A young man even, lured, seduced, sometimes on his first try begins to violate all the laws of nature.

But if reason and humanity, still reigning from the bottom of his heart, should prevent him from abandoning himself to the barbarous pleasure of pro-

---

[8]Original footnote: It seems that the most revolting disorders should be the distinguishing mark of the most enlightened of centuries. Consider the picture that *Petronius* paints of that shameless *Quartilla's* conduct in the world's capital. *Encolpe* and *Ascylte* are at *Quartilla's* house with Giton: after the two profligates had grown tired of the lascivious and revolting caresses, *Psyche*, a servant of *Quartilla*, approaches and whispers into the ear of her mistress. She responds: "Yes, yes, that's a good idea; why not? It's the best occasion one can find to make *Pannichis* lose her virginity." They made that young girl come immediately, who was exceptionally pretty, and who did not appear a day older than seven: it was the same person who had, a little earlier, entered our room with Quartilla. All those present applauded that proposition; and to satisfy everyone's eagerness, the necessary orders for marriage were given. "For me," it is Encolpe who speaks, "I remained unmoved and stunned, and I assured them that Giton had too much modesty to submit to such a test, and that the little girl was not old enough to endure what women suffer on those occasions." "What!" retorted Quartilla, "was I any older, when I made my first sacrifice to Venus? May Juno punish me if I remember ever having been a virgin: for I was merely a child when I besmirched myself with others my same age; and as I grew older, I diverted myself with persons older than myself, until I had arrived at the age I have now. I believe that it's about this that that proverb says: *Quæ tulerit vitulum, illa potest & toller taurum.*

faning the rosebuds before Zephyr's warm breath has opened them, he will soon see appearing before his eyes all that Nature has made most perfect. It is a young object, whose beauty causes tragedy: barely three lusters later, a burgeoning bosom, and still fresh; a rose and lily complexion... Nonchalantly reclining on a bergère, the goddess has chosen a posture most appropriate for showing off her charms; snow is not as white as the amorous deshabille that covers her; too short a skirt, a little bit disarranged, shows off half of her tapering leg; softly resting on a cushion, a pretty little foot entices a kiss, while the other falls negligently on the parquet; the seductive siren gives to her breast, which a containing corset presses, clinging to her slender waist, that lively and repeated movement that in a naïve beauty is the precursor of defeat: the Graces will open her cute little mouth; under two barriers of coral, ivory and pearl are glimpsed; her voice more gratifying than that of the lyre is heard; an arm, a hand, white like milk, extends, she makes a sign to the victim to approach; the soul is unsettled by that enchanting movement, one does not recognize himself anymore; the imprudent young man advances: already he's drunk on her voluptuousness; tumultuous desires stir up his blood something awful, and Beauty itself strokes him. Perfidious beauty, which knows how to appear tender – what am I saying? She will act the picture of modesty, only to give herself later, with an affected passion, when blind transports of feeling succeed timorous fears... O miserable young man stop!... stop! a serpent is hidden beneath the flowers.[9]

Alas! a view from the precipice is not strong enough to retain him: seduced by his heart, by nature even, and by his temperament, he rushes to his ruin. Ah! if only he knew the danger!... impotent wishes! he must pay for his slowly-acquired intelligence with the most precious good after virtue: his health.

The laws of society, decency, modesty, and above all adornment, stoke the desires, have become the principle secret of modern Prostitution: thus one will always see intemperate and sensual men, as long as delicacies and fine liquors agreeably tickle a gourmet palate: it is our laws' responsibility then not to destroy that vile state, for it will endure as long as they exist, but to diminish the inconveniences and dangers of it, which are physical at first and, by indirect consequence, moral.

Prostitution has not, in all honesty, produced the shameful contagion that desolates the universe; but it propagates it. It is the reservoir of it, the impure and constantly renewing source.[10] If guilty parties alone were punished by the dreadful consequences of a brutal sensuousness, the justice of punishment would not prevent this from always being a great evil for the human race... But, O wise mothers, you, who for so many years cultivate with care those tender

---

[9]Original footnote: They are not always so dangerous. See *Note A*.

[10]Original footnote: Although that terrible malady is accompanied by symptoms less serious than in the past, one must not think that they will ever go away by themselves.

flowers, the ornament of the fatherland, and nature's works of art; who, by your examples and lessons, inspire in your daughters love of virtue and a chaste decency; what bitter tears he prepares for you, that young spouse you destine for them! Blinded by factitious virtues, seduced by external brilliants, you are very far from imagining that he carries corruption and death in his bosom; he does not suspect it himself perhaps; and soon a young, timid wife, tormented by the poison whose nature and source she ignores, will perish doubtless, by giving birth to an innocent being, unfortunate like herself, who will follow her to the grave!

Yes, Prostitution is a necessary evil, everywhere where some modesty reigns; I am in agreement with all the universe and all the centuries: Sparta,[11] where that virtue was proscribed, is the only place in the world that I know of where one had not seen those miserable souls, whom ordinarily all vices band together to precipitate to the last degree of abasement

---

[11]Original footnote: The laws of Lycurgus make one believe that that legislator did not consider pudor as the preserver of chastity. The *girls* of Sparta were always indecently clothed: there are even occasions on which they appeared entirely naked in public, in order to compete among themselves in a race for the prize. "But by proscribing pudor, it does not demonstrate that Lycurgus had succeeded in preserving chastity; one of those virtues is the inseparable guardian of the other. The Lacedaemonians did not possess an irreproachable reputation, and among the vices that that nation is most often accused of, their libertinage was not forgotten."

> *Cantet... libidinosæ*
> *Lædeas Lacedemonis palestras.*
> *– Martial, Epig. 2 L. IV.*

and turpitude (A).[12]

A man who, as both a politician and a philosopher, visited all the places of debauchery in that Capital (with the precaution however of having, like victorious Roman Generals, someone always at his side charged with reminding him at every moment that he is a feeble mortal); such a man, I say, would be everywhere revolted, on seeing the grown, pretty girls, who, of all the advantages of their sex, lacked only mores, lost to society, to which they would have given robust, well constituted children, and of pleasant face. "Debauchery devours then whatever is most beautiful and most able to please," he would tell himself, just as war destroys the strongest and the tallest. It follows necessarily that the number of beautiful people must insensibly be diminished, and that they who would have a face and a figure must be vainer, more sottish, and more exposed to seduction. Perhaps you will consider, my dear friend, what I advance here as doubtful and destitute of proofs; but cast a glance on that multitude of almost-hideous faces, which inundate our cities; see the ugliness and the small or defective sizes propagate from father to son, from mother to daughter. Nature does not work like this. Observe countries where the finer sex is not im-

---

It remains to be seen whether *Lycurgus* did not regard *public chastity* as more harmful than necessary, in the State he wished to form. I make a distinction between *privato chastity* and *public chastity*; the momentary disorders of individuals can have an effect on the first, but never the laws, which have an influence only on the second.

[12]Original scholium: (A) the notes marked by capital letters are contained in the second part.

mediately snatched up but recognized, and in which the daughter of a peasant however beautiful she may be is destined for the son of a peasant; you will find that children inherit the traits of those who brought them into the world. I will go even further; mores contribute to beauty. Parents who lead a soft life must needs beget debile children, whose delicate hue and tender skin are not proof against the atmosphere and years; one also sees that in Paris, where one wants precocious fruits, precocious talents, precocious beauties, where everything is pre-ripened, overwrought Nature serves man according to his taste: the pretty children in their two sexes are not rare: but their traits grow ugly as they develop; the fine and brilliant color of those charming dolls resembles the superficial taste of the people; it is a flower that appears at its dawn with some splendor and pizzazz, but which withers before noon. On the contrary, I have seen in certain provinces, half-drawn faces, minds nothing less than penetrating, having arrived at adolescence, to astonish either by the regularity of their traits, or by the solidity of their genius. Yes, my friend, the human race has lost its attractiveness; here, by particular causes that I have just explained to you; in all parts of the world, by the mixing of peoples. The half-Tartar Persian, corrects, it is said, his natural ugliness, by mixing his blood with that of the beautiful Slaves of *Teflis*:[13] but the children are less beautiful than if they came from a father and a mother nourished in the fertile countrysides that the Kura waters, and than if those new offshoots had received the influence of the graces' climate. The Georgian himself, by depriving himself of

---

[13]Teflis: Tbilisi, Georgia.

what he has that is most perfect, does he not diminish the beauty of his blood? I do not believe that one can doubt it. We have then in the world more than half beauties; where they are found to be perfect, they are in the distant cantons of great cities, where reign, with the innocence of mores, an honest affluence: for misery deforms the body. Its fatal effects reach the soul, and *remove half its virtue*. Nothing easier, while going through the provinces, than to convince oneself of the truth I'm advancing. The poor wretches are always ugly; in the long run, abundance and equality would bring back the Charities, Venus, and the Graces. While waiting, pretty people will always be in such small numbers that one must forgive them their affectation. But who does not know that the poison from the Antilles irreparably undermines the human form?... What more powerful motives can be imagined in order to bring us to desire than that we should put some order in a condition that appears in truth little suited to being regulated, but which used to be in the past, and which nothing prevents from being again:[14] Life, the health of its citizens; our daughters' best interest, whom their wisdom does not shelter from a malady that one cannot admit being affected by without blushing; the attractiveness of a face, beauty, the second advantage of humankind, which many regard as the first!

But that is not all: one could obtain from the

---

[14]Original footnote: Prostitutes were left to fend for themselves, at around the time when it was most necessary for them to be watched over by a wise administration, i.e., on the arrival of *syphilis* into Europe.

places of Debauchery, when put in good order, a real advantage. It is what I will develop in the following Letters; for this one is already too long. You do not like those fastidious Epistles that contain merely sterile phrases: I hope to satisfy you according to your taste, by submitting for your examination some ideas that can be of some utility for the human race.

* * *

EVEN THOUGH your lovely wife writes to you also, she wants me to pass on to you her warm and friendly greetings and also those of the beautiful Ursule. I salute you, my good friend, and am, with an inexpressible pleasure,

– Your dear D'ALAZAN.

Fourth Letter

From the same.

May 3.

I have met with the charming Ursule twice, since my last missive, my dear friend; the first time, two days ago. Madame Des Tianges was with us; the second, today, and we were alone... Yes, alone. Does that surprise you? Eh, well, to augment your surprise even more, I will tell you that we spoke for nearly one hour together, and that I told her the most... surprising things. For instead of speaking with her about the only thing I might wish to discuss, I did not have the audacity to mention a word about it. In all honesty, that adorable girl intimidates me. She makes the petulant, the impudent D'Alzan modest and reserved; and then I also have to tell you that we were in the parlor. Madame Des Tianges had asked me to inform Ursule that she would stop by in the evening, to accompany her to a relative's house, whom the charming sister did not know. My dear Mistress (who does not yet suspect that I give her with all my heart so sweet a name) asked me about that Lady, her character, her beauty. The conversation would have ended immediately, for I hadn't a whole lot to tell her; but I did like *Pindar*, who, when the dull individual who was paying him to celebrate his victory in the Olympic Games didn't offer him brilliant enough material, praised Castor and Pollux – extremely adroitly, I turned the subject of conversation to Adélaïde Des Tianges; praise of her heart, of her mind, gushed from the source; I spoke for a long time and with warmth about her affection for you; I painted a picture of her pure mores, and I said something about her beauty. My eyes were fixed on the lovely Recluse, when I praised the graces of your spouse; and I will confess to you that, while using the name of Adelaïde, it was the portrait of Ursule that I painted. She must have realized it, for she grew prodigiously red in the face. This evening, I must accompany them. Conceive for yourself, my friend, how happy I will be! I will spend three hours at least with Ursule; it is while waiting for that desired instant that I write to you now. I return to the topic of my Plan.

Continuation

Section I. Necessity of Places of Prostitution

You have seen that my design is not to make Prostitution seen as absolutely intolerable in a well-regulated State: far from it; I consider it to be an unfortunate but absolute necessity in large cities, and above all in those miniature universes that one calls Paris, London, Rome, &c.

I recall having advanced that, among the ancients, Sparta alone must have gone without prostitutes. Lycurgus' laws removed, it is said, pudor from chastity itself, and from then on the desires must have been less violent.[15] But it was not enough: that Legislator, whom Greece regarded for a long time as the wisest of all men, knew the human heart too well not to sense that so long as a woman would be interdicted from all others except her husband, that powerlessness to possess her legitimately would suffice to make desire for her grow. He wanted his citizens, among whom everything was already held in common, to be able to make requests of each other, and to lend each other his wife. He imposed even the obligation on any man, who could not have children with his own wife, to cede her for a time to another. In a republic where all citizens were equal and ate communally; where by consequence the luxury of cuisine, clothing, buildings were impossible, unnecessary, or ridiculous; where the same man finally could lay claim to all beauties, and women could follow their inclinations which the laws did not reprove,[16] Prostitution, that vilifying condition, which lowers a charming girl to a position in-

---

[15]Original footnote: "Love could have produced great ravages, principally among a people moved to enthusiasm: severe laws, multiple obstacles, would have served perhaps only to make it more dangerous: *Lycurgus* took a completely opposite approach; independently of exercises in which the girls were entirely naked, he wanted that their ordinary clothes should leave them half naked. He forbade celibacy under pain of infamy, allowed husbands to lend their wives, and authorized men to borrow the most beautiful women, addressing themselves to their husbands. All those laws, while attacking faithfulness and pudor, removed from love almost everything there is of delicacy and seduction; but at the same time, they weakened that passion, and guarded against the furies of jealousy." – *Dissertation by M. Mathon de la Cour, on the causes and degrees of decadence in the laws of Lycurgus, crowned by the Academy of Inscriptions and Belle-Lettres*, 1767.

ferior to the beasts even, must not have and could not have existed.

In Athens, in Rome, and in the rest of the universe, where the mores were much less exact on the article of marriages, such as they exist among us today, there were places of Debauchery. But I am persuaded that the number of prostitutes in merely the city of Paris or London surpasses what might be found in Greece or all of Italy, at the time of the greatest corruption among the Greeks or the Romans: because, besides divorce which was permitted, a master had the right to make his Slaves satisfy his pleasures.[17] That is even the reason that, in our days, there are almost no Mussulman prostitutes, very few among

---

[16]Original footnote: Here is how a Lacedaemonian responded to the man who asked him, "*In Sparta, what was the punishment for adultery?*" -- that *the guilty party was obliged to give a bull tall enough to drink from the top of Mount Taygetus in* Eurotas. "*But,*" said the questioner, "*it is impossible to find such a bull.*" "*No more impossible than to find an adulterer in Sparta.*" In effect, what constitutes a crime is opposition to the laws: all crimes against society, so severely and so justly punished, would be nothing more than indifferent actions, if society was dissolved. One also knows that the Fathers of the Church, deceived by the Lacedaemonian's response, quite often cited to Christians the example of Sparta's women. One has to admit that they could not have made a worse choice. See the previous note.

[17]Original footnote: *jus primae noctis*, which certain lesser *Vaudois* lords still enjoyed one hundred fifty years ago, was a leftover of that barbarous custom. The *landowner* among those nobles, consequent to their rights of domain, bore the right *of deflowering the bride on the first day of nuptials, and possessing her on the first night*. All the enlightenment that had been spread throughout Europe with the rebirth of philosophy was needed to make those little tyrants blush, for a so-called right that had been almost widespread, under the Christian empire even.

the Indians and inhabitants of the New World.[18] The two hateful types of impudicity, which the barbarous Spaniards accused those latter people of, so as to give a shadow of justice to their massacres, to their tyranny that was crueler than death, was so much calumny, which the pious Bishop Las Casas,[19] who had traveled widely throughout South America, justified.

Far be it from me the thought of proscribing pudor, excusing divorce, and seeking to diminish the just horror that the barbarous usage of buying a beautiful girl inspires; as if that treasure, greater than all the riches of Monarchs, could have a price placed on it, and as if the despotic empire that is placed over her in that way were not as contrary to nature as it is to the lights of reason. Our mores, as dissolute or dysfunctional as they appear, are preferable to those of the Ancients and Muslims.[20] I dare say more: it would be better that we saw prostitutes grow in number, and that our wives ceased to be surrounded by a swarm of contemptible seducers each day. In so hard a condition, would that they could all, faithful like the charming Adelaïde Des Tianges, never introduce into our families children who usurp our rights and steal our name! Experience teaches us that a wife who has forgotten herself to the point of failing in her first duties, never stops there: maternal love disappears in an adulterous soul; sometimes property is dissipated, in order to pay for the expenses of a vile *procator*;[21] and often a husband of good faith does not leave his long

---

[18]Original scholium: see *Note A*.

[19]Original footnote: Las Casas was Bishop of La Chiapa in New Spain.

security except ruined and betrayed. But to seduce a woman, an honorable girl, one must make an effort, take pains, and sometimes dispense enormous sums; for the fairer sex digs a large hole beneath us, which swallows up not just the property of the man she dupes, but that of the lover she favors. I have seen, my dear Des Tianges, many contemptible men, for whom crime is a game, be scared away by the consequences of an intrigue and abandon it; they would prefer one of those women, whose profession is something worse than gallantry, because, so they say,

[20]Original footnote: Those who wish to advocate the virtues of the *Turks* and almost all the Asiatics in general are free to do so; for me, I consider the men of those countries as nothing but cowardly slaves, who avenge themselves basely on the feebler sex. They are not husbands, they are disdainful masters, or jealous tyrants. What country is that, good God! where the man buys the object of his love at the fair! No, he who thinks he is able to buy and sell his equal, and who regards it as an allowed act to destroy another human being without killing him or her, cannot possess an idea of true virtue. Those rather famous *Chinese* who, it is said, in even the basest of conditions, assist each other civilly, or dispute amongst themselves the honor of ceding in circumstances, whereas carriage drivers in Paris or London pull on each other's hair; those vaunted Chinese drown their daughters when they believe they have too many of them; not to mention their craftiness, and other faults, that the *Voyage of Lord Anson* has revealed. Fortunate Europe, keep your virtues, even your vices, rather than envy anything from those climates!

[21]Original footnote: Our language lacks a proper term to render this idea; I thought myself permitted to borrow a phrase from the mother tongue of our own language: *Procus*, from the ancient Latin verb *procare* (to ask insolently) and figuratively (cajole another man's wife) is the proper term, which I render with *procator*. One makes do with the word *adulterer*, but other than this word being the same for the crime as for the criminal, the lover of a woman is not always her *adulterer*.

they are without consequence, and one leaves them or gets back together with them when one wishes. And if they did not find one? It was the end for them: they would have sacrificed everything they owned to satisfy the first of passions. I concluded from this that Prostitution is an evil that makes us avoid an even greater one.

Effectively, in our present state of mores, and in a century in which the number of Single People is so greatly increased; when one sees even those who are engaged in marriage forming a criminal plot of living only for themselves, and afraid to leave a posterity;[22] when Ecclesiastics have so little enthusiasm for their profession (because in fact there are few men who could have it[23]), what is the virtue that could be sustained over a long period of time against a slew of enemies bent on its destruction? The laws, even the

---

[22]Original footnote: This crime is not particular to our century: the Roman wife named *Pannicus* took culpable precautions against pregnancy:

> *Cur tantum euneuchos habeat tua Gallia quæris,*
> *Pannice? vult f... Gallia, nec parere.*
> — Martial, *Epig.* 67, Book VI.

[23]Original footnote: The author of the *Dissertation on the Laws of Sparta* makes this sensical remark: "Laws perfectly conformant with humanity would assume a new strength every day, instead of undermining and weakening others little by little over time, and sooner or later finishing by abolishing them." In fact, to order for men to do what they cannot act on except with great effort and continual internal combats is to prescribe for them what they will never do, or not do for long. Every effort that tends to lift a man above his nature is honesty's pitfall; for a man cannot be sustained except by the enthusiasm of novelty; it produces hypocrites consequently: a type of dishonest people, the most dangerous of all.

most severe, would they have enough strength to protect from violence a sex that glorifies giving birth to peril, but which fears participating in it? A crowd of Strangers inundates large cities; have left their acquaintances and their mistresses; but their desires follow them: they are aroused at the first object they see, all the more facile given that the fair sex of the Capitals is the most seductive, the most coquette; to make matters worse, the sudden privation in which those Strangers find themselves, from their ordinary amusements, leaves a void in their heart, which makes them totally vulnerable to love. You may fill in, my dear friend, the gaps. Eh! how many seductions, abductions, rapes, Prostitution allows men to avoid! Imagine taking a more difficult, not to mention impractical, route; imagine changing our mores to the point that commerce ceases almost entirely between the two sexes; what will happen then? An even greater evil: loathsome *catamites* will impudently brave the laws and nature; our children will be exposed to all the indignities of a brutal passion.[24] [25]

* * *

Madame Des Tianges comes to remind me: we are going to pick up Ursule. Take care of yourself, my good friend. I am your very devoted,

    — D'ALZAN.

---

[24]Original scholium: [See Note] B.

[25]Prescient.

Fifth Letter

From the same.

May 15.

Ah! my dear Des Tianges! That instant waited for with so much impatience, it has passed... and I would still like to be desiring it. Ursule did not receive the confession I had made of my feelings as I had hoped. I have never desired her presence more ardorously. Would I happen to have a rival? Has someone else already touched that heart of hers, the possession of which excites all my desires?... Ah! Des Tianges, how miserable I would be!

I was beside that proud beauty; we were given some freedom to speak; I did not lose so favorable an opportunity to open my heart. Ursule heard me out; but with a coldness capable of disconcerting a man less amorous than myself. No, if her heart were free, she could not have prevented herself from being softened by all that I said to her. Madame Des Tianges shares my sorrow; she feels sorry for me; but alas! if her adorable sister is insensible to me... that thought overwhelms me and follows me everywhere I go. I do not know any remedy for it, dear Des Tianges. If you saw at present that capricious, that fickle, D'Alzan, that madman, who braved a sex he is not worthy of adoring; who denigrated it, mocked it, contemned it; who judged it only by the Prostitutes he haunted, and his own corruption; if you saw him humiliated, weeping... I know your heart; it would be touched, penetrated. Could you not, my dear friend, hasten the decision of affairs that detain you, and come back quickly... But Ursule, would she love me any more? How fortunate you are, Des Tianges! If my fate could one day resemble yours! Ah! I have known neither happiness, nor pleasure even: to enjoy life, one must be loved by an honest, charming woman; and that good which is so great, what have I done to deserve it?

I will continue today to converse with you about my Plan, as much to distract myself, I must admit, as to acquit myself of my promise: one must give to one's friends things only that have value. If I wrote to a man of prejudice, to one of those purists who help themselves to the least peccadilloes of poor men, I would not have explained myself with so much candidness on the Necessity of places of Prostitution. I would fear, with reason, to be considered, in the mind of such a man, as one of those Epicureans who lacks mores, who might wish to be able to abandon himself to his criminal penchants in complete safety. I have no reason to fear that injustice from you, my dear friend; and the dispositions that I show today are a sure guarantee that I am a changed man.

Section II. The Inconveniences of Prostitution

No, my dear friend, I am not at all blinded to the inconveniences of the *publicness* of a certain number of women, even with the reform that I would desire be introduced. They are still very great. For example, I cannot stop admitting to myself that, firstly, if one regulated places of infamy, it would seem thereby that the Government was giving them an attention they little merited.[26] Secondly, that sure, facile, rather inexpensive pleasures would procure the satisfaction of an illegitimate passion; would diminish perhaps the number of honest unions.[27] Thirdly, that a Christian must not regard it as a thing of little import, the crime that my Plan cannot help but favor.[28] Fourthly, and finally, that some people will be able to believe that the type of approbation one gave to lost women would affect mores, by accustoming society insensibly to look with less contempt on this latest period of human perversity.[29] Which also, nearly, echos in summary form the observations I read in your letter on my proposed system. I do not speak to what you add to that: *That it*

---

[26]Original footnote: This objection, the strongest and most sensible of all, will no longer cause embarrassment if one directs one's attention to all the precautions that the Rules have prescribed, making Prostitution entirely different from what we see it to be today. Moreover, the evil is so great, that one must resort to poisons even, if it might result in salutary effects. I will say it again, the evil is so great, that one must not be delicate in the means used to diminish it.

[27]Original footnote: The first inconvenience is real: this second one appears to me unfounded: honest men who are well-off will not get married any the less, just because there is a *public place*: country folk, whose numbers are so important to our State, will hardly think to go there. There will be, then, only our libertines and our voluntary bachelors; and those men, as one knows, are already lost as far as the country is concerned. The Establishment can only shrink the gap that the deregulation of our mores has left.

[28]Original footnote: A Christian knows that God draws good from evil even. Alas! and we humans, we often draw evil from good!

disarms divine justice, which punishes the impudicity of that very life, by chastisements that are born from the disorder to which debauchees abandon themselves. You didn't recall that I had anticipated this objection.

Let us examine now that throng of dangers that we avoid, by exposing ourselves to four inconveniences which exist, even today, independently of my Plan.

Firstly, *the dreadful malady that Prostitution spreads and propagates uninterruptedly, continuously*. Its ravages are spread over multiple generations, without individuals having been imbued by a new *virus*: the mineral that is employed, the regime that is observed, weakens the temperament: a leaven that art never succeeds entirely in destroying attacks the principal viscera, above all the stomach and the lungs: there is no complete recovery; the *economic animal*, very strongly shaken, never resumes a perfect equilibrium again. If the guilty parties were the only ones affected by that cruel evil, one could regard it as a just punishment for their disorders; but their children are also involved. I said it at the beginning, tender and unfortunate victims are seen to become prey to an evil that is all the more dangerous as they do not suspect even having been touched by it: it has already made irreparable damages, by the time one recognizes the symptoms that belong to it: the newborn and their wet nurses perish miserably. Humanity and reason sug-

---

[29]Original footnote: This idea will no longer persist once we have sufficiently penetrated the motive behind the establishment of *Parthénions* in the first place.

gest that one must neglect nothing to protect and save those innocent creatures.[30]

Secondly, *a throng of young women, almost all of them pretty, the nation's best in terms of shapeliness and constitution, are lost to the fatherland.* One knows that in that condition, as dangerous and as humiliating and painful as it is, they rarely reach the midpoint of their career. Debauchees of all stripes abridge the course of their life. They do not give back to the STATE the tribute of work each of its members owes it; they spend their miserable days in a kind of numbness, which they do not exit from for the most part until evening when they lay their traps wherein the wisest of men are caught sometimes as well as the libertine.[31] The fatherland, deprived of the subjects whom all those girls might give it, girls who consider pregnancy to be the greatest of misfortunes; not because it makes them produce ordinarily unhealthy children, who perish immediately, or live infirm lives; but because it always causes an irreparable setback to their attractions. Also, they employ all imaginable artifices to avoid pregnancy, or to procure an abortion, on the first sign of pregnancy.

---

[30]Original footnote: Lots of people are occupied with searching for sure and easy ways to cure *Venereal diseases*, without resorting to mercury which is incommodious and dangerous: the so-called discoveries can all the more enrich some Charlatans, whom the secret of procuring palliative cures makes famous; but the Government can dry up the source; it holds in its hands the most powerful of antidotes. See *Note A.*

[31]Original footnote: One kills a rabid dog and serpent as soon as they are found; are they, physically even, as dangerous as a *public woman*?

Thirdly, *places of debauchery, distributed as they are among us, often give rise to, for certain women,[32] the design and occasion of eventually indulging in a vile penchant for libertinage, which they would not have given in to if there had not been a means for satisfying it. Young women, too dominated by a preference for adornment, seduced by the attraction of gain, sometimes led by temperament,[33] go to those places to lose their innocence and their health; their good, but inattentive parents thus become the dupes of the confidence they placed in their children.*

Fourthly, *all the disorders reigning ordinarily in places of Prostitution.* The evil would be less, if only the natural penchant were followed there; but those who draw the line on that could almost be considered wise. Besides, the natural route would not be the surest; and, in spite of himself, a man is constrained to indulge his depraved tastes. He is assured that he will not find any resistance, the girls needing to accept all manner of act, which exposes them to the same dangers as men, as well as to what is particular to them and what they fear so greatly, which is pregnancy. There is then no genre of degradation that those poor souls do not endure: they are seen to abandon themselves to what is most repugnant to them, either for interest, or for fear of being mistreated, something the most loathsome complacencies do not allow them always to avoid.[34] Love, that divine feeling that

---

[32]Original scholium: See *Note C.*

[33]Original scholium: See *Note D.*

[34]Original scholium: See *Note E.*

the Supreme Being makes grow in our hearts to disseminate there a sweet inebriation, which allows us to support the miseries of life and consoles us in the saddest expectation of death;[35] love, I say, when it is not accompanied by esteem, turns a man into a ferocious animal; it is love without esteem that makes him more furious, crueler than anger even![36] he satisfies himself while gnashing his teeth, and harms what he just caressed!

Fifthly, *accustomed to seeing immodest women, men's contempt for them comes down on an entire enchanting sex; whom,* I finally recognize, my dear friend, that *we cannot render homage to, without glory redounding to ourselves.* Will I say it? those graces, which are even more so when half-veiled, no longer excite in our heart that trouble, that delicious quivering sensation, the first, and perhaps the sweetest, of pleasures. When, consequently, by pudor, a chaste wife steps back from their transports, men are incapable of knowing the price of a modest reserve. They teach their virtuous companion, – they demand from her, – those shameless caresses that debauchery has turned into an art.[37] Madmen! they do not realize that love and beauty are tender flowers that wither as soon as they are touched, that dry up when too-avid a hand wants to press them!

Sixthly, *a great drawback that results when public women, or even kept women, live among hon-*

---

[35]Original scholium: See *Note F.*

[36]Original scholium: See *Note G.*

[37]Original scholium: See *Note H.*

est citizens is that one can see, and often sees, what goes on in their rooms. If a young man, a young person, has unfortunately discovered a place in their home that allows him to be instructed on what goes on inside a house of prostitution; what a baneful change presumably that dangerous view will have on his or her mores! Your daughter's imagination will be sullied; the imprint it makes on her fresh soul will never go away perhaps. And your son? He himself will soon want to become familiar with what he only caught a glimpse of. Often, also, the upper floors of a building, the first floor of which is occupied by public women, is inhabited by common folk of honest behavior; their wives and their daughters on returning home will find themselves exposed to discourses, to fondlings... They will need to lodge elsewhere, and humiliated virtue gives way to vice.

Seventhly, *lost women go outside, promenade, some make themselves noticed by the elegance of their attire and, more often yet, by the indecency with which they expose their seductive charms; imprudent young people take, even in public, criminal liberties with them.* And our children, witnesses often to those horrors, swallow the poison; they ferment, they develop with age, and that dangerous sight leads them to their ruin, despite the efforts of a vigilant father or mother. The daughter of an artisan, of a bourgeois even, at that age, when native ingenuity does not make her suspect anything amiss, sees a welldressed woman, whom young military men track, accost, caress; that innocent girl feels growing in her heart a desire – weak, it is true, but it will grow stronger, – to be like them, and it will pave the way to disorders one day perhaps.

Eighthly, *in a Public Garden where the senses have just been affected by all that the Capital has to offer of the most seductive kind, one meets objects similar to those one has just desired.* To escape the peril, one must have a virtue tempered by every test, or lack the temperament. But what indecency! which children dispersed throughout the Garden are exposed to... when, hiding under the cover of a half-obscurity, one dares... And people are surprised at the corruption of mores at the earliest ages!... Knowledge of pleasure precedes predilection and usage.

Ninthly, *often a public woman tired of the capital, or fearing the vengeance of those to whom she has transmitted the poison that circulates in her veins, or even other crimes making her redoubt the magistrate and the laws, goes elsewhere to spread her contagion.* It is then that, exhibiting libertinage and villainous indecency, one sees her scandalize the public vehicles where she is found.[38] People of all ages, lacking in mores, gather round her; one hears dirty and disgusting songs echoing, the revolting phrases of a coarse brutality. Woe to young people lacking in experience who are witnesses to the thousand infamous scenes that those miserable wretches occasion. It is enough sometimes to make them lose their innocence; woe, above all, to ever-curious young women, whose attention, despite themselves, will be fixed on scenes unseen until then: vice is so contagious that the example, which should frighten, often diminishes the horror that one has of it.

---

[38]Original footnote: This happens particularly on water transports.

At other times (and in this case the peril is nearly inevitable), one runs into public women who disguise themselves under a modest and reserved attitude. The most scrupulous decency accompanies their discourse and their manners; a seductive and modest negligee repairs the decay and ruin of their attractions; an honest man sees them: his heart speaks to him on their behalf; he becomes obliging, complaisant, filled with considerations; he is touched by several remarks of gratitude; he is moved; a seductive smile succeeds finally in charming him: his principles abandon him (eh! who can resist the coquetry of a woman whom one believes to be honest!). Night falls; they get close to one another; the occasion, the senses, sometimes the heart... a man is so soon taken!... the obscurity... he takes advantage of it to savor a dangerous kiss from an impure mouth... he grows bold... the resistance is imperceptibly nuanced... he succumbs... and the honest man, seduced, pays with his health, sometimes with his life, for the momentary forgetfulness of his duties.[39]

If the Prostitute, along the way, can cause all those ravages, what disorders will follow her on arrival in a countryside village, among men whose inexperience makes them facile to fool; whom the thirst for illicit pleasures devours; thirst that the *seasoned* attractions in the style of large cities kindle even more?

I content myself with merely touching on these principal sources of crime that Prostitution, such as it is endured, occasions every day. The Prince is

---

[39]Original scholium: See *Note I.*

the image of Divinity; like it, he knows how to draw good from evil even: he alone could give life to an Establishment, which I draw up a plan of, that I believe would be easy to put into practice. That precious advantage, to make particular abuses contribute to the general wellbeing, is the most glorious appanage of Kings.

Adieu, my dear Des Tianges: may your swift return make it such that this letter is the last you will receive from Your good friend

– D'ALZAN.

P.S. We received your Letters, just now. "*When Monsieur D'Alzan attacks, one really must surrender!*" You mock your friend, Des Tianges; and you should feel bad: the charming Adelaïde knows the bounds of friendship better.

Sixth Letter

From the same.

May 24.

Listen to this, my dear Des Tianges; I have just overheard a secret, and I confide it to you: the *divine* Ursule... forgive me the expression; I don't know if it is strong enough: eh well, that charming girl has come this morning to see your wife. I arrived an instant later. Old Jeanneton, whom I have the good fortune of not displeasing, and who seeks to secure for me all the pleasures that are in her power, the old Jeanneton, your cook, whispered into my ear, before having announced me. I was able to control my eagerness; I passed into your study, not to spend some time there managing our affairs, according to my habit since your absence, but with the design of reflecting for a moment on what I needed to say to the proud Beauty who captivates me. I found nothing that satisfied me: I abandoned myself to the saddest thoughts. – There you have it, then, I said to myself, that D'ALZAN, whom no one could resist; whom the too vaunted merit of a seductive face made so vain; that presumptuous man who for the longest time believed that all women aspired to the conquest of his heart; behold the man; he founders... before a child!... Those *very moral* reflexions set out on a tone to carry me far away, when Madame Des Tianges, and her charming sister, came into your room. I didn't want to show myself immediately, and did well not to do so, for I became the subject of conversation. O! my friend, that Adelaïde, whom I believed to be close, so naïve, so good, how fine she is!... She felt sorry for me the other day, with so honest, so touched an attitude... Here she was saying to her sister: "Men esteem the conquest of our heart only in proportion to the trouble it costs them, my dear Ursule: whatever the feelings that Monsieur D'Alzan has inspired in you, you must not be false, but employ a wise dissimulation. He has merit clearly, and I prefer him to all others for you, my good friend; but for that very reason, I want to assure myself that you will both be happy: I want to have solid proof that his tenderness is not a blind feeling, a passing fancy, that would not withstand the trial of marriage; and I have good reasons to think that. Let me guide you, my ever so dear sister, your happiness is as dear to me as my own. I do not find it strange that Monsieur D'Alzan should please you; I would have a wrong opinion of your heart if it was insensible to the merit that a thousand agreeable talents and graces accompany, in a man whom we destine for you, who loves you, who has told you so: but there are characters whom a certain type of woman have ruined... one must distrust all lovers. Yours is a man of honor, but... there is a fickleness. Do not count on him, and do not abandon your heart to the sweetness of being loved, except when I tell you, *it is time...*" I was on the verge of coming out of the study, and getting down on my knees before Ursule, to convince her by the vivacity of my transports, and by the most sacred oaths, of the truth and duration of my love. Ah! Des Tianges! I swear on the bosom of amity, I love, I love forever... I was afraid to displease them, by showing myself. Your wife continued: "Not all men are like Monsieur Des Tianges; they do not all have that true character that one untangles at first sight; not all have mores as pure as his... Not that I wish to make you listen to... ah! my dear, it is a happiness similar to the one I enjoy with respect to the most estimable of men, which I seek to procure for you, by uniting you to my husband's friend; but let us not neglect anything that human prudence prescribes: I desire, as much as you do, and more vividly perhaps, that your lover should be worthy of a heart such as your own; of that so tender, so pure heart, that my own responds to. To tell you the truth, I think that Monsieur D'Alzan will be amenable to the counsels of his friend; that he will follow his examples; I see in their humors a rapport that makes me conceive of that flattering hope; but he is still quite young yet, men don't have reason until they are thirty years old; you, you are barely out of childhood... let's wait, my dear friend; let's wait a while; there is no need to hurry; I would be almost as loath to cause Monsieur D'Alzan a misfortune as you."

"My tender sister," responded Ursule, "I sense all the wisdom of your counsels, and you will never see me deviate from them: I have let you read into the innermost recesses of my heart; deign to act as my mother; heaven, for a long time now, has deprived us of her who cherished us; you alone have felt that loss; you always make every effort to make it up to me. O my sister! my dear sister! Ursule will never stop having for you all the tenderness of a submissive daughter."

They embraced each other, my dear Des

Tianges; I saw them; I could barely contain myself: for several moments, they hugged each other... O my friend, art is nothing in comparison: how could it do justice to that divine model! I was going, I believe, to show myself, but they had left; and I am happy for it; for I am delighted they do not know that I overheard them; I want to leave them the pleasure of following the plan that they have traced out; I promise them complete success!... What adorable women! Des Tianges... Adelaïde!... divine Adelaïde, how worthy you are to be Ursule's sister, and the wife of my friend!

I am happy, my dear friend: you can sense how much I must be... After a while, I presented myself to Madame Des Tianges, after having advised the good Jeanneton to keep our secret. Adelaïde received me with an open attitude; on her face, and in her manners, I could see an attractive candor, joined to an attitude of affection for me, which deeply touched me. My charming mistress, true to her sister's advice, was polite, but nothing more. As for me, what I had just heard, cast over all my exterior an air of liveliness, the vivacity of which I was not always the master of moderating, despite my desire to do so. I affected from time to time to fix on the portrait of Madame Des Tianges, and on that of Ursule, who for several days embellished your wife's apartments; and from the corner of my eye, I glanced at her lovely sister; I noticed with satisfaction at that time that her beautiful eyes were fixed on me; but when I raised mine, hers looked elsewhere. Adelaïde was obliged to leave us for a moment, to attend to some business; as soon as I found myself alone with Ursule, I assumed that submissive posture that so pleases beautiful women, and the only one I might desire for over an hour: I painted a picture of my feelings at the knees of the incomparable Ursule. I glimpsed her efforts to hide from me her distress, her extreme agitation; despite the rigor she endeavored to arm her glances with, – her eyes were tender: she told me to get up, and she did not think to withdraw her hand, which I was covering with kisses; when she realized this, she put on so sweet an attitude that I renewed my misdeed a thousand times on the both of them. Can you conceive, my dear man, in what a delicious state of being I found myself in? Sure to be loved by the most beautiful, by the most virtuous, of all girls; sure that her heart, with the intelligence I had, shared my felicity, I saw in her modest resistance only the efforts of her virtue. Ah! that there was the pleasure after which my heart was sighing for so long without knowing it; Ursule is the first to make me enjoy it. From now on, I will be insensible to all others. To love an estimable object, to be loved in return, that there is joy; one takes pleasure even in the rigors of an adored mistress.

Madame Des Tianges returned, when I was still at her sister's knees. I did not change my posture at all: I renewed before her the oaths I had just made to the lovely Ursule, that I would adore her forever. I urged the beautiful Adelaïde to speak in my favor, to say something about my sincerity. "I would be more than happy to," she said to me, while taking both my hands, so as to oblige me to follow her into another room; "and if I can believe my presentiments, I will do so; but, my dear D'Alzan, I tremble for my sister;

her character is of a sweet melancholy; when her heart is touched, she will love too much; I would rather that she did not know yet, so soon, that passion, which will make her of all women the most to be pitied if she does not procure a complete felicity... Examine your heart thoroughly then, my dear D'Alzan, before telling her that you love her; in the end, she would believe you, and all your life you would have to reproach yourself for having deceived her."

She did not want me to respond, my good friend; she said that they had some business to attend to; we returned to Ursule, and I was dismissed, while she reminded me that today was the day I was supposed to write to you; but she added that she was expecting me in the early evening.

I obeyed, my dear friend: steel yourself with patience; I will put before your eyes a Rule, not like that of the Abbey de Thélème,[40] but a sensible plan, which would diminish the dangers of Prostitution, and which would compensate as much as *possible* by a real utility the abuses that one cannot entirely avoid.

---

[40]Original scholium: See *Note K*.

Section III. Means of Diminishing the Inconveniences of Prostitution: Lessons that One Can Draw From a Well-Run Public House

It is said that in Rome, public women are under the protection of the State.[41] But without going to find examples from among foreigners, it is certain that the French Government formerly did not consider that object as too vile to fix its attention on.[42] Our Monarchs themselves would give, to *Ribalds* or to *public women*, Letters of safeguard. Not, in truth, in order to favor those vile people; but so that the protection of the laws might prevent someone from committing in their houses a number of the horrors reported in the notes to my last letter.[43] The Magistrates and the inhabitants of the cities of *Narbonne, Toulouse, Beaucaire, Avignon, Troyes*, &c. included among their prerogatives the faculty of having a *red-light* district, or public house of Prostitution, of which they were the administrators. A misunderstood zeal for religion is, as far as I know, the only reason for the change that has happened in that regard amongst us. The devotees of a narrow-minded genius are enthusiasts; they follow without discretion the movements of their bile and take them for divine inspiration; they have falsely

---

[41]Original scholium: See *Note A.*

[42]Original scholium: See *Note L.*

[43]Original footnote: See *Notes C, D, E, G, H*; in the second part.

imagined that by proscribing debauchery that debauchery should be eliminated. What happened instead? They destroyed the remedy, and the evil has subsisted.[44]

It has always appeared to me that by placing things on an ancient footing, and also by giving to the new Establishment a degree of perfection that would result from its usefulness for the State, we would see a number of disorders disappear; we would avoid the shameful maladies that have ravaged the human race for so long a time, principally in Europe; and the sweetest and most noble natural penchant would be less debased.

Love! Love! How the times have changed! In the past, men erected temples to you; incense, the sweetest perfumes, veiled your altars with the whirlings of their precious vapors: today in the mud, ignored, despised, brutal *Lubricity* has snatched away your quiver, your bow; and as for your arrows, it has snapped them in two, all those that inspired a tender attachment merely. On your throne, cold *Insensibility* is seen, which madmen have mistaken for *Virtue*. What hand, friend of humanity, will pull you up out of the mud, o Love! and give you back your temple and your altars, chase out the *girl* from the *Furies*, unmask false *Virtue*, and make this consoling truth resound through all the universe: *Mortals, happiness awaits you on the bosom of your beautiful companions: it is Love, Love alone, that will give it to you!*

---

[44]Original scholium: See *Note A*.

Plan of Rules

For PUBLIC WOMEN in consequence of the establishment of Parthénions,[45] under Government protection.

Articles

I
Houses

It would be appropriate to select one or more houses, convenient and not too flashy, where today's Public Women, of all ages, will be obliged to go, under pain of corporal punishment. Those who continued to lodge them would be cracked down on and given a stiff penalty, without any regard to the reasons they allege by way of exculpation. Their informer, whoever it might be, would be recompensed by a portion of the penalty, which will be remitted immediately after conviction.

II
Kept women

One will distinguish from among lost women, those who are kept by a single man: it is believed to be necessary to tolerate them because otherwise that would

---

[45]Original footnote: *Παρθενείς*, conclaves of virgins, or girls. This word is clearly poorly suited; but those that would be more suitable, *πορνο**** in Greek, *Lupanar* in Latin, *B**** in French, might have offended delicate ears.

be an attempt on the freedom of citizens: but the least scandal on the part of those women would cause them to be led to the *Parthénion*. Kept women will be obliged to practice more decency than ordinary women because they will be taken away on the first complaint made against them.

III
New houses

Since the Establishment will be able to provide for this expense, new houses will be constructed that will be clean and proper, as laid out in Articles X and XIV. New subjects will be housed there, whose lifestyle will be regulated as one will see in what follows.

IV
Administrators

There will be, to govern the *Parthénion,* a *Council,* composed of twelve Citizens of perfect probity, who will have been honored with Aldermanry in the city of Paris; with the Capitoulat, or the quality of Mayor, in other large cities: they will have below them, in order to govern in the house, women, whose youth, to be honest, will have been spent in disorder; but in whom one will have recognized ability, gentleness, and who will have none of the defects incompatible with the position they fill. Those women will receive each day, from the Superior, sums necessary for the maintenance of the girls, and for interior reparations: they will give an exact account of their expenses.

V
Term of office

Each Administrator will be in charge for six years; so that after the first six years, two new administrators will be elected every year; and every year the two longest in office will leave their charge. They will give an account of their term in office, before the Tribunal appointed by the Sovereign, two months later.

To avoid the abuse that Administrators could practice by their authority, each Governess will have a list of sums that she will ensure are placed in the Depot during the day,[46] that no Administrator can ask to see; and the Superior will give those notes, every evening, to the Assistant Clerk of the Tribunal before whom the accounts must be rendered; and if that Assistant prevaricated by suffering someone to see the notes, he will be severely punished.

No Administrator will be able to enter into the house during its operation, neither as Administrator, nor in unofficial capacity asking for a girl, on pain of dishonorable and shameful discharge from the Administrative Body.

Taxes normally imposed on Administrators, for all types of tribute, will devolve on fellow citizens during the time of their employment.

VI
Subjects to be received

---

[46]Original footnote: see the last disposition of article XVI.

Young women who present themselves, when the Establishment is set up, must be received without inquiries made as to their family: far from it, it will be expressly forbidden by the Administrators for Governesses to inform themselves, and for the girls even to confide in their companions, about their family: but one will be extremely scrupulous in the examination of their health. Whatever malady they might be afflicted with, it will not serve as a reason to refuse them; they will be treated and cured; and if the malady should be incurable, they will be considered *Outmoded*, and their fate will be governed by article XLI: no one older than twenty-five years of age will be accepted.

VII
Asylum of the *Parthénion*

The *Parthénion* will be an inviolable asylum: parents will be unable to take their daughter out despite their relationship: they will be unable to speak to her even, if she refuses: and in the case where they are introduced into the house, under the pretext of asking for her as one of the girls, they will be escorted out as soon as they have been found out.

VIII
Mistakes

The Governesses will be unable to inflict any punishments: they will have the right only to make their report: they will be unable even to employ too strong a reprimand: they may only exhort a girl to do better the next time. When a girl will have caused some disturbance, or committed some grave error, she will be led into a room adjoining the one where the Administrators gather, whom the Governesses will have informed beforehand, not at all being allowed to appear with her, or to accuse her to her face: then the Council of Administrators will enter into the room where the guilty girl has been left alone; they will hear her defense; and provided she raises some doubt in their mind, they will remit her as if she had entirely justified herself, after having given her some advice and remonstrances. If the girl is absolutely at fault, they will always demonstrate a great disposition for clemency; at a first and second offense, they will content themselves by mentioning the punishment, and only the absolutely recalcitrant girls will be punished.[47]

IX
Crimes

If some girl becomes guilty of a serious crime, for instance destroying the fruit that she carried in her womb, she will be locked up in prison for one entire year, and given only bread and water. If a man has counseled her to abort, he will be punished according to the ordinary laws.

---

[47]Original footnote: It might be feared that so great an indulgence would degenerate into abuse, if the Rules didn't anticipate it.

X
Location of *Parthénions*

The houses of prostitution that are to be constructed will be located in sparsely populated neighborhoods: they will have a Courtyard and two Gardens: the only windows that will give onto the Courtyard will be those of the Governesses and those of *the children of the house*, whom article XXXVIII will treat of. Everyone, without distinction, will enter through the courtyard. There will be two sentinels at the gate to the first Garden, entry into which will be forbidden to women and children: all men indifferently and of every condition will be admitted into that Garden: they will find different entrances there, marked by the trees, bosquets, and trellises, to allow for slipping in without calling attention to themselves, into places where Bureaus similar to those at the Theater will be found; they will be quoted a fixed price by Tariff, while receiving a Ticket, which will designate the Corridor, and which side of the Corridor the man who received it will choose [a girl]; so the ticket will be marked with the number of the Corridor followed by the numbers 1 or 2, as will be seen in article XVII. The girls' windows will give onto the Gardens, but they will always be garnished with awnings, over the first garden, in such a way that they can see out but that nobody can see in. Next to the gate to that Garden, there will be another much smaller gate, always open, and placed in such a way that one accesses it secretly; it will be guarded on the inside by a Governess, who will only allow entry to women. It is through there that the girls will enter who want to enlist in the *Parthénion*; they will be received, at whatever hour of the day they present themselves, night or day. The second Garden will be for the girls and the Governessess' exclusive use; the public, and even the children born in the house, who are destined for work, will never enter there.

XI
Manner of presenting oneself at the bureaus

It will be permitted to present oneself masked at the door to the Bureau, where one will be obliged to remove the mask, in order to be seen by the Governess, who hands out the tickets only. One can go masked even as far as the entry of the Corridor that one chooses, where one will be obliged to leave the mask with the Governess who opens the door and takes the ticket.

XII
Man's choice

As soon as a man is in the Corridor designated by his Ticket, a Governess will lead him into a small, dark room; she will raise a small sliding panel, or *guichet*, and the man will examine through that opening all the young women on the right or left side of the Corridor, gathered in the communal hall designated for them; he will make it known to the Governess which one among them he chooses; and that Governess, after having led the man to the young woman's room, will go find her.

XIII
Girl's choice

When a girl is chosen, and the Governess has led her to the room that she is used to occupy, the girl, before entering, will enjoy the same privilege as the man had who asked for her; that is to say, she will examine him, by opening the *guichet*, which will be in the door of each room; and if she refuses to enter, he will be obliged to make another choice, without the girl being obliged to tell the reason for her repugnance: but she will not return immediately into the communal hall, in order to hide from her companions their knowledge of her refusal.

A man who, because of old age or ugliness, is constantly refused by the girl of his choice, will be given the opportunity to choose a number; a choice will be made from among the girls in the communal hall; for example, if there are one hundred girls, he will give any number whatsoever, between *one* and *one hundred:* the Governess will then go into the room; she will ask each girl to choose a number; and whoever chooses the number that the man has written down on the piece of paper, the Governess will make her go and find him right away.

XIV
Guardroom

Beside the Office, there will be a Guardroom, but it will not have a view onto those who take the Tickets. The guard's job will be to maintain good order on the outside of the house; to assign sentinels to various posts, and to act as a strongman, on the Governesses' behalf, whenever the need arises. To that end, there will be a bell in the Guardroom, with rope pulls in each of the Bureaus, so that on the slightest noise or disturbance, the Governess can alert the Guards; severe punishment, and in accordance with ancient Ordinances, will be administered to all those who wish to disturb the tranquility that must be maintained in the house, without regard to rank or dignity, which latter will be held as null and void in these places.

XV
No weapons

Each Guest will hand over to the Governess his cane, his sword, or his mask; the Bureaus will be furnished with a sufficient quantity of small armoires, all the compartments of which will be numbered, and a number engraved on a piece of ivory will be handed to each man, to recover the things he deposited there, before leaving.

XVI
Tickets

There will be different Tickets, according to the degree of youth or beauty. The girls will be lodged in the Corridors, in the following order:

The first Corridor, divided, like all the others, into two classes, will be occupied by older girls: their age will not exceed *thirty-six years*: those from *twenty-five* to *thirty* will occupy the second; in the third will be girls from *twenty* to *twenty-five*; one will find in the fourth, girls from *eighteen* to *twenty*; in the fifth, those from *sixteen* to *eighteen*; the small number of girls that could be found from *fourteen* to *sixteen* years of age, who will have developed at an early age a temperament that would allow them to receive men, will occupy the sixth Corridor. Girls younger than that, come on their own, or brought by their parents, and who will not have been deflowered, will be raised with care at the house's expense, by honest women, and they will not enter into the ranks of subjects at the *Parthénion,* when they reach the minimum age, except by choice. If they ask instead to learn a profession, they will be instructed, and they will be set up as children of the house, in conformance with what is prescribed in Article XXXVIII.

XVII
Tariff

Girls distinguished by greatest beauty will occupy the right side of the Corridor, marked by the number 1; the left side will be designated by number 2.

The Tariff for Tickets will be posted at the ticket window of each Bureau; the various prices will be on display there.

NOTICE

Girls chosen from among the *Outmoded*, who are discussed in article XXXIII, who are from *forty* to *forty-*

five years old, six sous, per...   0 liv, 6 s

Those from *thirty-six* to *forty*, twelve sous, per... 12 s

The First Corridor
No. 2. eighteen sous, per...   1 liv 8 s
No. 1. one livre, four sous, per...   1 liv, 4 s

The Second Corridor
No. 2. one livre, sixteen sous, per...   1 liv, 16 s
No. 1. two livres, eight sous, per...   2 liv, 8 s

The Third
No. 2. three livres, per...   3 liv, 0s
No. 1. three livres, twelve sous, per... 3 liv, 12 s

The Fourth
No. 2. four livres, sixteen sous, per... 4 liv, 16 s
No. 1. six livres, per...   6 liv, 0 s

The Fifth
No. 2. twelve livres, per...   12 liv
No. 1. twenty-four livres, per...   24 liv

The Sixth
ninety-six livres, per...   96 liv

This will be the income of the establishment. The Governesses will take turns managing the Bureaus; each person, on receiving a Ticket, will show them the money that he will give: the strongbox where he will place it will be constructed and behind bars, such that it cannot be removed; only the Governess will be able to slide it into an opening in the coffer by means of a stick attached to the box, one of whose ends will pass into the loge, and which the Administrators will have the key to; and the Governesses will immediately write the amount given on a sheet of paper, which will be sent to them every morning by the Assistant Clerk mentioned in Article V, and which they will return in the evening.

XVIII
Titular lovers

If a client, after having seen a girl, testifies that he loves her, and that he is content with paying the price of the Ticket to see her each day, that girl will be freed from having to gather in the communal hall, and no one else may ask for her. In the case where the girl would be of the sixth Corridor, the titular lover, in lieu of a charge, each day will give *twelve livres* only; *six livres* for a girl from the fifth, and so on, as long as her age brings a diminution. Girls from all other Corridors will follow the general rule.

Kept girls will be lodged in a separate building; their rooms will be disposed in such a way that communication from one to the other, and with the rest of the house, would be done only by introductive Governesses appointed to the task, who alone will have keys. Kept girls will be able to associate with each other; those girls will even have the liberty to spend time with the rest of their non-kept companions whenever the latter are not in the communal hall.

There will be a different Entrance for titular lovers, who will always be introduced by two Governesses.

Each man who choses a mistress, after having been assured of the girl's consent, will be led with her before the Head Governess; one will write before her, in a register, the *Parthénienne's* name and age only, with the No. of the apartment she must occupy; the titular lover will receive, on a morsel of ivory, that same name, with the No.; the Register, signed by the man and by the Superior, will be given back to the introductive Governesses, and put away by them in an armoire, under its No.; that Register will be unable to be seen, even by the Administrators, except on request of the titular lover.

A man who fails to pay or to show up after more than one week will lose his mistress.

In case of absence, one will alert the Superior, and one will deposit into her hands, either in money, or in guarantees, the agreed upon sum of money.

XIX
Prohibited marriages

The son of a well-to-do family, who has been taken with a violent passion for a girl whom he would be the first and only favorite of, will be unable to obtain her for a wife as long as he remains under his parent's authority or that of his guardian's: he will be unable even to make *sommations respectueuses*,[48] permitted

---

[48]*sommations respecteuses*: in French law, a juridical procedure by which two of-age children, a future husband and his wife, constrain their parents to accept their marriage.

under the Law, after having attained his majority at thirty years of age: but a man who is his own master will be heard, if it is determined that that marriage will not bring him too much prejudice; which request the Administrative Council will scrupulously examine. One will be very attentive to the mores and capabilities of people of low-extraction whom a *Subject*[49] of the house of prostitution consented to marry.

XX
Pregnancy of unkept girls

Girls, on the first sign of pregnancy, will occupy a portion of the house set aside for those who find themselves in that condition: they will be treated with particular attention. After these regular subjects of the house (those who have no titular lover) have given birth, the infants will be placed with a wet-nurse; but their mothers will take all the precautions they judge most effective to acknowledge them on their return to the house; and one will accord them the satisfaction of seeing their offspring once a week.

XXI
Pregnancy of kept girls

---

[49]Original footnote: There is a great difference between the *subjects* and the *children* of the house: the first have an indelible mark; the second may have all virtues and qualities; one knows too well that low birth does not deprive a person of virtues and qualities any more than illustrious birth provides them. Those difficulties, consequently, will not surface for girls born in the *Parthénion*, and who are destined for marriage, in the manner provided for in article XXXVIII.

When a kept girl is discovered to be in the condition described in the previous Article, if the father of the child she carries wants to look after his mistress, at his own expense, he will be permitted to do so: he will choose such person as he wants for the delivery, or he will accept those who work in the service of the house: he will be able to have the child taken away, or to have the mother breastfeed and take care of the child; to raise it secretly, or as his child; and in any case, he will not be obliged to instruct whomsoever it might be of its fate. He will be free to indicate it as the heir to his fortune, in the event that the man should die without legitimate heir or that he should be unable to contract marriage: he could also leave it to the care of the house, to be raised, and have it marked in a place on its body that is not apparent, and which cannot inconvenience the child: one will make mention of that mark, or of any other precaution taken by the father, in the *baptistery*, and the house will be obliged to hand over that child to its father on first request, without charge.

XXII
Communal halls

All the girls of a corridor will be assembled in two halls, with no. 1 or 2 marked on the doors, *eight* hours a day: scil., from *eleven o'clock* in the morning to *one o'clock* in the afternoon; from *four o'clock* to *seven;* and from *eight thirty* to *eleven thirty*, which will be suppertime. They are seated, tranquil, occupied with reading, or some work, as they choose; each place will be marked by a different flower, which will give a name to the girl who occupies it: thus, those whose place is designated by a rose, an amaranth, &c. will be called Rose, Amaranthe, Muguette, Narcissus. Each girl will always occupy the same place. In between those hours, and other exercises, and all the time that precedes *nine o'clock* in the morning, they will be free to take some fresh air in the second garden. Exempt from that rule, as with all those who are responsible for maintaining discipline, are those who have a titular lover, to whom they give all their attention, according to the conditions contained in Articles XVIII and XXIV.

XXIII
Exercise and meals

There will be set hours defined for the toilette and for meals: one will rise at *nine o'clock* at the latest; breakfast will immediately follow; the girls may occupy themselves until *eleven* by getting dressed and making themselves up; or if their toilette is completed earlier, they may dispose of the remainder of time as they fancy; as, for instance, visiting companions, taking a walk, &c. One will dine at *one o'clock*: from *two o'clock* to *four o'clock*, there is music and dance; at *seven o'clock*, a meal; a lesson on instruments until *eight thirty*. All the girls will be in bed by *one o'clock* in the morning, with no exception to the rule. The other hours of the day will be employed as prescribed in the previous Article.

Nights will be fixed at a double rate, in the first five Corridors: there will be no rate at all imposed in the sixth, unless it is for titular lovers.

No grief will come to those who keep to their room at the hour of lessons, and they will not even be reproached, if their absences are rare. Otherwise, the Governesses will gently bring up with them the error they make: if that was not useful, they will make a report to the Administrative Council. The penalty that the Administration can then dole out will be up to their prudence, and conformant with the spirit of gentleness recommended by Article VIII: but one feels that in an Establishment where chastisements are practically banished, some other resort is needed to replace them: those will be distinctions, and flattering recompenses, which will cost the house nothing, for those girls, for example, who make more marked progress in the arts that they are taught; it is what the measures contained in Article XL effectively tend toward. The surest means to prevent the girls from being refractory to measures in the present Article will be to make their Exercises fun, rather than a serious occupation, and the administration will succeed all the more as there are few women insensible to the pleasure of giving themselves an additional grace or of developing those they already have.

XXIV
Privileges of titular lovers

A lover who wishes to assign a particular teacher to the girl he loves, or who could himself teach in the mastery of music, dance, &c. will exempt her forever from having to appear at the house's lessons. He will be able also to exempt her from visiting the communal refectory in her Corridor, by providing for her board at his own expense; and in that case, eating with her and spending with her all the time he deems appropriate; as also making her remain in her room during her pregnancy, without other conditions as prescribed by Article XVIII and this one.

XXV
Employment of time in the communal hall

The girls will have instructive and amusing books given to them for the time they spend in the communal hall; those who wish to occupy themselves with work will be furnished with all they need; but there will be no die, cards, or any other kind of game in the communal hall.

XXVI
How often a girl can be asked for

The same girl will never be able to be chosen by different men on the same day; but if the same man asks for her again, one will permit the girl to go find him. No one will be admitted into the house before *nine o'clock* in the morning, except men already known by the girls, and who can ask for them by name.

XXVII
Frequency for an *Outmoded*

Girls of the third Classes will be exempt from the preceding article; those who for the most part are unable to have children any longer, and who will appear each day as many times as they deem appropriate; age, experience, and the heat of passions which have died down, leading one to believe that they will not abuse that privilege.

XXVIII
Infidelities

If a girl, loved[50] by a man, feigned to reciprocate his feelings in order to engage him to marry her, or merely to persuade him to make her a mother, and if she should deceive him, by receiving another man; as she would only be able to do when at least two Governesses were in the know; those who favored her will be punished grievously,[51] and the girl will be separated from the company of others and condemned to hard and continual labor for the rest of her days: only he whom she wanted to deceive can save her from that sad state.

XXIX
Board and other arrangements

The table will be served without profusion, but with a sort of delicacy; clothing will be in good taste,[52] and each girl will dress in the manner that best pleases her

---

[50]Original footnote: kept.

[51]Original footnote: by death.

and suits her. A lover who wishes to give to his mistress clothes of his choosing, and at his own expense, will be able to do so, as well as any other presents he judges appropriate; which will belong exclusively to the girl, without the *Parthénion* being able to claim anything more than the ordinary price of admission, which will always be received in advance: but in the case of the girl's death, without child, the house will take possession of everything that belonged to her.

The Governesses will treat the girls with consideration, care, graciousness, almost never letting them perceive the authority that they have over them. Their beds, linen, everything that will be at their disposal will be well-selected, clean, well-made, and comfortable. The Governesses will distribute and pick up their linen every other day. They will ensure that each girl, assisted by the *Visitors*, discussed in Article XXXIV, make her bed as soon as she has risen.

Everything contained in this Article will be observed for all classes of girl indifferently and without exception.

XXX
Expense for habits

There will be no uniformity of habits whatsoever; each girl will be provided for as prescribed in the preceding Article; but, in order to avoid too considerable expenses, a limit will be set on the amount employed for each girl's wardrobe; each girl will be free to dis-

---

[52]Original scholium: See *Note M*.

pose of that amount as she wishes, whether to spend it all on one outfit alone, or on many, each of which would cost less. However, the Governesses, to ensure that the girls are always exceptionally clean, will ensure that each has a sufficient number of outfits. As outfits are outgrown by the girls, or they no longer wish to wear them, they will be used by the children born in the house who are destined either for marriage, or for following in the footsteps of their mother, or to become laborers, and those outfits will be reworked to fit them; paying attention to give the most magnificent outfits to those of the two first classes.

XXXI
Baths[53]

There will be warm and cold baths in the house, and each girl will take one or the other of them every two days throughout the year: scil., in *summer*, warm and cold baths; in *winter*, warm only. The laborers themselves will be required to take a bath once a week in *winter*, and more often in *summer*.

---

[53]Original footnote: It would be desirable if this practice were followed in hospitals, above all those for children, as the *La Pitié*, the *Correction de Bicêtre*, and the *Enfans Bleus, Rouges*, &c., as baths, in those establishments, would prevent maladies of the skin which are common there, and which, if they don't kill the children, torment them, retarding or preventing their growth, impoverishing their temperament, &c. As for the *Parthénion*, warm baths are absolutely necessary for the girls who take little exercise; they will stand in for them, favoring thereby a suitable perspiration in them; they will keep the *girls* and *laborers* in a heightened state of cleanliness; their frequent use will diminish disagreeable odors that are detected in all places where many people are obliged to gather together continually.

XXXII
Cosmetics

The girls will be forbidden to have any scent at all; to put on blush or powder; to make use of creams to soften their skin, it being recognized that all those things give only a false shine and destroy natural beauty. Exempted from this rule, those who have a lover, they being at liberty to follow their predilection: but they will not be exempted from the rule of the bath: and the Governess will ensure that at minimum they take a bath in their room.

XXXIII
The *Outmoded*

The amount of money girls procure for the *Parthénion* each day, the daily expenses and necessities subtracted from that, will be put in reserve, to create a dowry fund for girls born in the house or who were received too young, and for taking care of the *Outmoded*, the maintenance of buildings, &c. One will choose among subjects *thirty-six* years old or older a certain number of girls who still retain some beauty, in order to compose the two first classes, who will be available for only *six* and *twelve* sous; so that all men of each estate will find the *Parthénion* girls at a rate proportional to their means, and will never resort to those miserable wretches who, having no fixed retreat, can brave the Laws and violate with impunity the rules of an exact policing; but so that *Outmoded* girls might conduct themselves with least repugnance to receive those who are located at the bottom rung, one will observe three things: the first, making them take a warm bath on entering; the second, that they remain with the girl only for a half hour; the third, that those who show up with a bellyful of wine, will be kept in the house until their drunkenness has dissipated; in that way, one will grant them what they ask for, either a girl, or their exit; and in the latter case even, one will not ask them for the price of admission.

XXXIV
VENERAL DISEASES

Visitors

The greatest attention will be employed to preserve the girls from that horrible malady that makes this Establishment so desirable: Governesses will be chosen from among the girls in whom both age and desire for pleasures have disappeared, those who will have always fulfilled their duties best, and who will be the most intelligent, so as to visit with the men who present themselves. They will allow them entry only into the Corridor that the their ticket designates, and only after they are assured that they enjoy perfect health. They will even visit the girls every day, when they rise; it will be like a novitiate of Governesses; those who acquit themselves of that employment to the satisfaction of the College of Governesses will be elected by them, provided vacancies are available.

XXXV
Head Governess or Superior

Each year the Administration will appoint a Head Governess, and she will always be from among the Governesses who will have distinguished themselves by their greater attention or prudence. She will have no other function than to ensure that each Governess is exact at her post: she will receive money for expenses; she will be present at the opening of the Coffers of Receipt, at the remittance of Notes by each Receiving Governess; but the most important of her duties will be to keep a continual eye on the manner in which the *Visitors* acquit themselves in their employment, and the care they take of girls who are pregnant, or in the case discussed in Article XXXVII.

XXXVI
Amends

Men who are afflicted by the illness discussed in Article XXXIV, and who will have had the imprudence to present themselves, will be obliged to pay a fine; and in the case where the guilty party lacks money, he will be obliged to pay the equivalent in jewels or effects, which he may have to sell in order to have the required sum: if the illness was, however, still rather unpronounced, so that one had reason to believe that the affected person was acting in good faith, the fine will be light, as for example double the price of admission.

XXXVII
Treatment of the girls

If, in spite of all these precautions, a girl finds herself incommoded, she will be sequestered on first indications, and she will not leave the infirmary until after a complete and perfect recovery: as the girls will be visited each day precisely, by those who compose the novitiate, nothing will be easier than to assess their condition; they will be examined even when they leave the bath. On the least indisposition that they experience, one will be attentive to ascertain the type: but no remedy will be administered, except on the advice of an able Surgeon attached to the house. That experienced practitioner will not acquit himself of his duty hastily, as those in our Hospitals do; his efforts will be recompensed by suitable honors, and by distinctions worthy of a man useful to the State. His entrance to any other part of the house than the Infirmary, except in cases of urgent and unexpected necessity, will be forbidden in the same manner as with the Administrators.

XXXVIII
FATE OF CHILDREN BORN IN THE HOUSE

Boys

So that the State might draw from the Establishment of the *Parthénions*, the utility of which was mentioned earlier, it will be observed firstly that girls will be prevented as much as possible from taking precautions against pregnancy; secondly, that the population of the house will be favored in every possible manner, above all in the maintenance of integrity, and, I dare say, pudor even, at the heart of incontinence and impudicity; thirdly, that one will dedicate an immense amount of attention to the children, from the moment they are born, until the age when they are discharged them from the house; fourthly, that all those not recognized by their father will be reputed children of the State and, as such, destined to serve it; that is to say, those who have a suitable constitution; fifthly, that one will make a first choice from among the boys who are *eight years old*: those who are well built shall be destined to compose a corps of troops that will be exercised from childhood and which, together with the Foundlings gathered from all the Hospitals in the Realm, could replace the peasant militias; sixthly, one will teach those young soldiers reading, writing, arithmetic, geometry, fortifications, and artillery service; there will be Teachers responsible for their education, taken from Royal Academies; those respectable Corps always have members, zealous for public wellbeing, who will consecrate themselves voluntarily for that work, without other motive than the honor they accrue; seventhly, the *Parthéniens* will serve for six years (from *sixteen* to *twenty-two years old*) in the corps of militia: at *twenty-two years old*, a second choice will be made from among all meritorious subjects, who will form a regiment of royal grenadiers, the which, by consequence, will be composed only of *Parthéniens*: they will remain there until *twenty-eight years of age*; there will be a third promotion from among those who are distinguished by their mores, intelligence, and bravery, and they will form a corps called the *Company of Merit*;[54] after having again proven their ability, after six new years of service, subjects drawn from that Company will be distributed among all the regiments, so as to give lessons of military art to the Soldiers; the most handsome men among them could have a much more noble destiny still, and replace the foreign guard around the sacred person of the monarch; those who should go that far would have the right to marry, after having obtained permission from their Commander; eighthly, as only a very small number of them would obtain that honorable post, the quality of *Military Master of Art*, and even entrance into the *Company of Merit*, the other *Royal Grenadiers*, having become veterans, will be recompensed according to their ability; on quitting the regiment, they may marry, and they would be assigned, in order to live and raise a family, to different posts in the Realm that should be held only by veterans; they would make up the Guards of public safety for the city of Paris, the Maréchaussées, &c. Those who, because of lack of intelligence, or some fault, are retained in the *Militia Corps*, will remain there as long as they are in a condition to serve; or, if they request it, they could be incorporated into different Corps, and in the Regiments of the provinces.

As for those who are valetudinarians, dis-

---

[54]Original footnote: It is natural that a man who is attached to nothing, like a bastard, should be more suitable than another for serving the State; that he would above all be more devoted to his master; for he will concentrate in it what other men distribute among their father, their family, and the State. There will not be, then, any post for which those good people are not worthy; no enterprise that cannot be entrusted to them; their loyalty, and their courage above all, will be unshakeable.

abled, or too short, one will assign them professions proportional to their forces; gentle and easy for those of the first and second type; they will become tailors, cobblers, weavers of silk and cloth for use by the *Parthénion*, which will sell at a profit what they produce in excess; the most robust among them will be placed in jobs requiring strength, like gardening or other labors necessary on the interior; but one would give the opportunity for rapid development to those who have genius; one would favor their dispositions, and their progress would determine their fate.

Girls

As well, a choice would be given to the GIRLS. Girls starting at the age of ten: firstly, one would set aside those who are poorly constituted, or ugly; they would be taught trades; the product of their work would be destined for the house, which would provide them with all that they needed. Those who would have defects other than ugliness, but who would be of a healthy temperament, would become producers of dresses or fashions that the girls could wear: they would learn how to dress the girls' hair, and everything that is necessary for their adornment: one would take care that they are instructed by the most able Female Teachers; and that the most becoming manner, best taste, and novelty will be incorporated into their labors. No foreigners, neither men nor women, will be employed in the service of the *Parthénion,* once there are children for the task.

Secondly, the young women born in the

house, who have a nice face or figure, will be at first instructed with special care: they will be taught in the different arts, such as *design, painting, dance, music, fashion,* and above all the *great art of adornment*: one will let them decide for themselves a trade: they will not at all be encouraged to take up the profession of their mothers; on the contrary, the honest education that they will be provided with will be suitable to inspire them to put some distance between themselves and the *Parthénion*. When they have decided to live in the world, they will be given the professions they indicated: one will encourage them to marry, with a dowry of *one thousand ecus*; observing to give their hand only to men of certain position, who have a standing, and property equal in amount to the girl's dowry, or a superior talent in their profession. The male children of the house, who can marry, will be preferred to all others, unless the young woman had made a selection before they were presented, or the competitor presented too considerable an advantage to the mistress not to be preferred.[55]

A particular outfit will not at all distinguish the children of the house, or those who could, in whatever manner it might be, be employed in its service.

---

[55]Original footnote: One could still choose, from among the two sexes of *Parthéniens*, subjects who would have the most agreeable face or figure, and who demonstrated the best disposition, in order to prepare them for the *Theatre:* the Administration would take precautions, so as to preserve the purity of their morals, which will be seen in a Plan that a *young person* proposes to give in the near future, and that will be a follow-up to this one.

XXXIX
The Council's authority over children of the house

The Administrative Council will have the authority over all subjects exiting the house, with the exception of Soldiers, while they are in active service. It will guard against husbands squandering the dowry, and all creditors will be made aware that the dowry of *Parthéniennes* is inalienable. If the wife should fail in her duty, the Council would advise to put things in order, by all suitable means, even while bringing the seducer before the Tribunals, which would punish him corporally according to the case, the gravity, and the circumstances of the offense. A husband who is of a completely disorderly conduct will be banned; the Administration will watch over the affairs of a girl who came from the *Parthénion* if she is not in a position to watch over herself; the husband will be severely punished if he has been found to have treated her badly, that he had disparaged or disdained his companion, or that he obliged her to endure the indignities of a rival, &c.

XL
Selection of Governesses

The position of Governess will be proposed as a recompense for reasonable behavior; and it will be the expectation of those who, not having ever incurred chastisements or punishments of any sort, will be found to have the necessary intelligence and talent. One will prefer, for that employment, all things being equal, *kept girls*. They will have the right to exit, on days when their internal employment permits, on house business, or for some other reason, while notifying the Superior: over and above the consideration that Governesses will enjoy, there will be an attractive benefit attached to that position, which is that they will be able to have their children, those who are unrecognized by the father, married, according to their predilection, thus giving them a family name: and if they should not have any children, they will be free to adopt a boy or girl from among those of the house who please them, to see them united, to make them beneficiaries of their will, by giving them even a family name, and passing on to them all their savings. Those same rights, for young women's children, will be held by the Administration.

XLI
Fate of the *Outmoded*

The *Outmoded* who are unable to be employed as prescribed by article XXXIII, and the preceding article, will enjoy the rest of their days in a tranquil life, in a section of the house set aside for them: they will be engaged to occupy themselves, by recompensing them for their effort; but they will not be constrained.

If some one from among them had profited well enough from the exercises given to the girls, so as to find herself in a position to teach *dance*, *music*, and how to *play* some *instrument*, she would be employed by the house. Those *Mistresses* would enjoy a consideration proportionate to their merit; they would sit at the table with the Governesses, and they would have, like them, the privilege of leaving the house at certain hours.

XLII
Enclosure

The girls, once entered, will never leave, unless one of the cases mentioned in Articles XIX, XL, XLI, or XLIV should apply to them, or they have become heirs: the latter can go to manage their possessions, unless they prefer to enjoy their revenue by remaining at the house. The *Parthénion* will not receive any donation of goods from those girls, nor from any other persons. The heirs who have exited will remain forever under the authority of the Council of Administration, which will look after them, and make them return to the *Parthénion* if their conduct should become scandalous or dissolute.

XLIII
Girls who would want to change their life

A young woman, whose soul, after her entrance into the house, would be lifted by the decency of her exercises, and who would design to live as an honorable girl from then on, will be encouraged by the Council in that good resolution. The Administration will act as her parents, or will reconcile her with her own, after which she will be tested as to the sincerity of her resolution, so that they can be convinced that she may be permitted to call them as such: in a word, they will grant her all the good offices that reason and humanity will prescribe.

XLIV
The Parthénion when closed

The *Parthénion* will be closed on the principal festivals of the year: on those days, there will always be a play put on in the Theaters of the Capital, and a portion of the girls will be brought there; the carriages that will lead them there will be entirely closed; and the loges they occupy, furnished with a curtain of gauze, will be drawn before they appear.

XLV
Community among Parthénions

Administration of the revenue generated from all the *Parthénions* in the Realm will be shared commonly among the houses. Subjects will be able to go from one to another, according the prudence that Administrators believe necessary, &c., but the Administration of Paris will have overall authority and can, depending on the case, require that Subjects from houses of other cities be sent to it: with the exception however of kept girls, who are covered in Articles XVIII, XXIV, and XXIX, who will never change houses except in the case where their lovers went to live in a city that had a *Parthénion:* in which case, they must follow.

Such would be, in broad strokes, my dear Des

Tianges, the Rules of an Establishment that the physical and moral ravages of Prostitution would make necessary; which would doubtless do honor to wisdom and to humanity, which would prescribe their practice, and from which we would reap the benefits, which are greater and more invaluable than at first imagined. As you know, nothing is vile for *Gods* and *Kings*; from the moment that an object has utility, one glance from them ennobles it. The most abject cares are not the least important; it is with manure and mud that we enrich our gardens and our arable fields; see the *Polianthes tuberosa*, the Ranunculus, that rare tulip, – it is not Flora, it is a little compost that gives them their rich colors and all those treasures that we admire.

Good night, my friend; this Rule has occupied me so long that I am quite afraid the hour has passed when I might still visit with Ursule and your spouse... But no, it is not yet seven o'clock, and I am not expected until sometime before eight... Do not spare me your objections to what I send you: I will be much obliged if you could point out something I have not foreseen.

Love me, my dear Des Tianges, just as tenderly as you will always be loved by your *scatterbrained*, but faithful,

– D'ALZAN

Seventh Letter

Response from Des Tianges to D'Alzan.

Poitiers, June 1, 176*.

In two weeks I will embrace you, my good friend: I will enjoy my dear Adelaïde's presence, and yours; I will see your happiness, and that of Ursule; you are both, after Adelaïde, what I love most in the world. What happiness, my friend, to be the spouse of a wife for whom one feels the most tender love, and whom one esteems even more than one loves! That there in a nutshell are my feelings for Madame Des Tianges. She is still for me that charming bride (and she always will be), what Ursule is today for the passionate D'Alzan. Yes, my friend, your love for my wife's sister, completes my dearest expectation: I hope that you will be the felicity of that so sweet, so deserving, so beautiful girl; she will be yours, be sure of it, if honesty, a sensible soul, flattering consideration, a nice cheerfulness, – in a word, if all the solid qualities that one might desire in a companion have some sway over the heart of an honest man; I have known her for a long time, and I can answer for her. I have no offensive doubts about your constancy, your sincerity, your change of behavior; by giving my wife to you as your only society, at the time of my departure, it was, I hope, to prove to you my esteem and my confidence better than vain words could do. D'Alzan is already virtuous, because he desires to become so. My friend, we are going to live in such sweet intimacy! that is what I have always desired. For, why hide it from you: My dear friend, from the moment I married Mademoiselle *de Roselle*, I destined her sister for you. Love and friendship have seconded my views sooner than I dared flatter myself. You love each other; you were both in love at first sight! I accept, O heaven! so favorable an augur, which justifies the impatience I feel for the moment when, in my best friend, I will embrace my brother.

I will expend vain efforts to express to you all the satisfaction that your feelings have given me, the certitude of seeing Madame Des Tianges soon, and the happy success of the efforts I owe to my pupils. Although I write to my wife, as well as to the *divine* Ursule, inform them of my return first thing, if possible; for one receives deliveries a half hour earlier in your neighborhood, than in ours; fly to my house, as soon as you have opened my letter.

I do not wish to wait until I have arrived in Paris to speak with you about your *Rules*; because I am delighted still to receive here the responses that you intend doubtless to give to my objections.

I have read, I have weighed, with the most scrupulous attention, each of your Articles; and it is not yet at the point where I don't encounter infelicities. Without speaking about the Plan per se, I pass over to the dispositions of the Rule. Will execution of the *first Article* be easy, you think? and why does the *Second* remove kept girls? The *Third* requests something useful from the Establishment, which, as a result, will be more distinct, more separate, more sure, and less scandalous; but to build an edifice, expressly for lost girls, expedient, etc.! I don't know if it is quite proper that Échevins, Capitouls, &c., should be Administrators of those houses, as *Article four* desires? Your Governesses will they be sufficiently dignant to govern? Why forbid, in *Five*, Administrators' entrance into the house? I think I can guess the reason. What is the point of *Six* and *Seven*? *Eight* surprises me, and I don't see on what it is based, nor *Nine* for that matter. As for *Ten*, here's what I think: it is to virtue, and not to libertinage, that one must dedicate all these facilities. Eleven, same thing. *Twelve* and *Thirteen*: I see an problem in the second of those Articles, it's that the choice will be sometimes quite long, and that often it will end by the abuse one hoped to avoid, the constraint. *Fourteen, Fifteen*, and *Sixteen*: I say nothing about the first two; the *sixteenth* is a little shocking. Why such young girls? *Seventeen*, why are the fifth and sixth corridors put at such a high price? *Eighteen:* finally some girls who will not be public? *Nineteen*: despite your clauses, this Article could occasion some abuses. There will be some madmen who marry a public girl, who later repent their decision, and will be unhappy. *Twenty* and *Twenty-one*: all that diminishes the expense of the house: but that those children should become considerable legatees, that is not legal. *Twenty-two* and *Twenty-three*: the girls will be well educated, well dressed, well behaved! *Twenty-four*: those titular Lovers, to whose account you return often, will have quite the privileges! *Twenty-five*: fine; but will they abide? *Twenty-six* and *Twenty-seven*: the first part is good; but those poor Outmoded ones, how you employ them, mister legislator! *Twenty-eight*: oh! oh! now there's some rigor for you! *Twenty-nine*: you turn soft again immediately: I have my doubts; you have stepped out of character. *Thirty*: obviously you have your reasons for all that, but I'll overlook that Article; there is some economy there, and, without being greedy, I like it. *Thirty-one* and *Thirty-two*: pass again, but you seriously contradict the common practice. *Thirty-three*: what this Article requires is it really so necessary? Prove it to me. *Thirty-four, Thirty-five, Thirty-six*, and *Thirty-seven*: a fine! that would be quite well deserved, and the poor litigants have sometimes paid them, who were not, for the most part, so legitimate. I have nothing to say about the other Articles; they are necessary. *Thirty-eight*: ah! and now for some politics. But the revenues from your *Parthénion,* will they suffice to raise so many children? to marry them? to give the pretty girls dowries? *Thirty-nine*: good enough. *Forty* and *Forty-one*: I repeat, the Demoiselles will be in truth quite well treated! *Forty-two*: fine. *Forty-three*: now that's an excellent Article. *Forty-four*: they will benefit from those days of freedom to go to the Theater. I think, as you want to say, my dear friend, that the inhabitants of London would do better to go to *Drury Lane*,[56] on Sundays, than to get drunk on punch, and very expensive bad wine, in their taverns, where often young Englishmen forget their reason, and, what is worse, their innocence. *Forty-five*: Paris will be the administrative center, the residence of order's President.

That review is short. I would have made it longer, if I said everything I think, but more detail would take up more time than I can give to it; I owe

---

[56]Original scholium: Theater of London.

my time to my pupils. Rather, send me a response to these objections that each of the Articles has given rise to, as I have done, which are reduced almost to nothing. To tell you the truth, I think that if ever one wanted to regulate disorder, one could not pass up putting your ideas into practice. It would diminish the evil, and, thereby even, effect some good.

Hoc sustinete, majus ne veniat malum.[57]

D'Alzan! ah, instead, why aren't all men reasonable? They would seek an honest companion; they would find happiness, by making themselves loved, by loving in turn. What a sad happiness one enjoys in the arms of a stranger, by whom one is not even sure that, in the very moment, one is not hated, detested!... But, as the poet says:

Nitimur in vetitum, semper cupimusque negata;
Sic interdictis imminet æger aquis.[58] [59]

I know perfectly well that it is not possible for everyone to tie the knot... It is the calamity of the times, the shame of public Administration... My friend, I am happy; you will be too; or rather, you already are, the two sisters will be the felicity of two friends; let us bless the Supreme Being for them, and be worthy of the duration of our innocent pleasures, by leading a pure life, and above all by engaging in

---

[57]Original scholium: Phaedrus, fab. 2.

[58]Original scholium: Ovid III. *Amor.* El. 4-w. 17-18.

[59]The original scholium attributes this phrase to Ovid ("the poet"), but it appears to be from the Bible, Proverbs, 9:17: "Stolen waters are sweet, and bread eaten in secret is pleasant."

beneficence towards our fellow man; that there is, have no doubt about it, the most agreeable act of grace in the eyes of the Father of men. No, D'Alzan, it is not difficult to be a good man living at leisure. What horrible ingratitude it would be if we violated the laws of society, we who are its favorites! We fulfill a duty, we work for ourselves, when we are the stay of those less fortunate than ourselves, the model and the consolation of other men; the aid that we procure for them binds them to us; the example of our virtues is the rampart of our assurance and security. What would become of us if people who have nothing to lose learnt, from those whose fate they envy, how to brave divine and human Laws!... Goodbye for now, my dear brother: tell your Ursule for me that, after her sister and yourself, I merit being what she loves best.

— DES TIANGES

Eighth Letter

Reply from D'Alzan to Des Tianges.

Paris, June 16, 176*.

Good Des Tianges! I did not think it possible to love you more; you call me your brother, my respectable friend, and you speak to me with a cordiality worthy of that quality that you ascribe to me. Your friendship does not resemble those ancient liaisons in which I prostituted that sacred name; with you it is a sincere attachment, so tender and durable that it penetrates me with gratitude, and convinces me more and more that there is joy only in virtue; the virtue that makes you love me, that gives me your sage advice, that supports my sometimes impertinent repartees, and that destines for me the sister of the adorable Adelaïde, when I was so little worthy of her!...

From the moment your Letter was received, I flew to Madame Des Tianges': I present it to her; she reads two words, and makes cries for joy: – "I will see him again then," she repeated completely transported! "in several days time we will be together again! Oh! we will not leave each other's side again; I promise." She called everyone in your house together, your old lackey, the good Jeanneton, your assistants, and even the little Negro: "Monsieur Des Tianges is on the point of returning, my dear children," she said to them; "in less than two weeks time from Poitiers; you are going to see your best friend again." I didn't understand what everyone responded as they were all talking at once; they made a deafening sound; but their faces shined with joy; your old lackey, with tears in his eyes, ran to your apartment to put everything in order to receive you; and lady Jeanneton, looking twenty years younger, made everyone in your household dance with her.

The package for your wife and for Ursule arrived at that same moment. A profound silence ensued; Madame Des Tianges had the kindness to read aloud a portion of your Letter; your entire household gave evidence of an extreme sensibility to the memory you honor it with. We immediately made preparations, Adelaïde and I, to carry your delicious epistle to Ursule... My what sweet things you know how to write! In all honesty, if it weren't for the kind things you said about me to my mistress, I would be jealous, but really very jealous. After having read, and reread, the two sisters conversed together privately for several instants; I do not know yet what they said to each other: Ursule blushed; Madame Des Tianges caressed her; I watched them, and I found myself happy.

She is still reserved around me, my good friend: on the evening of that happy day when I penetrated Ursule's secret, that secret of a tender heart, which it is so sweet to surprise, we supped at the rich and boisterous B**'s house... A thing that will revolt you, as much as it surprised me, is that in an honest gathering of very well-chosen guests, he had not thought that the impudent D*** was out of place... You know how magnificent B** is: in order to make the regale complete, he had arranged everything so that a superb ball should complete the celebrations that he throws for one week now: but that ball was a mystery; our colleague seasons the pleasures that he procures with something of a surprise. He had taken the trouble to find dominoes[60] for the Ladies; they appeared delighted: everyone of them put on a different disguise. They did a thousand crazy things; they teased us, they tickled us; pretended feelings, naïvety; and escaped as soon as they read in the eyes of their dupe that he was tempted to take their little pleasantry seriously. D*** tormented me a great deal; I did what I could to avoid her; for it was not hard to guess who she was. I was all the more concerned when I had lost sight of my two dear companions. Madame Des Tianges and her sister, so as not to stand out, masked themselves like the rest. They had the mischief not to reveal themselves: I looked for them anxiously: they played on my embarrassment, and apparently wanted to see what I would resolve to do: but when, in my agitation, they judged that the masked lady who obstinately followed me was wearing my patience thin, that boredom was gaining the upper hand on me, and that I appeared completely cold to those pleasures that formerly were so much to my liking, Adelaïde approached me. She made an effort to disguise her voice, but I recognized her immediately; my joy appeared so natural and vivid to her that she was touched: she led me to her sister. I danced with my dear Ursule: ah! my friend! how charming she was! if I had not adored her already, at that moment she would have made a conquest of my heart. We withdrew to the side finally, and we were chatting, when

---

[60]dominoes: a half mask that covers the eyes.

that accursed D*** came to mix with us. She had the audacity to hold a thousand words with me, which were only clear to me, but which caused me a great deal of anxiety all the same. Happily, someone came to take her away to dance, and that other person (who was none other than B**) not abandoning her anymore, we were left alone until five o'clock, when we were separated. Our conversation filled me with a thousand charms: we spoke of you; I expressed my feelings; she appeared to listen to me with pleasure; Adelaïde, from time to time, pressed her sister's hand; there was a moment when I thought I saw Ursule's beautiful eyes moistening with tears; the movement of her bosom was more pronounced... Also, at that moment my expressions were so tender, I felt so strongly what I said, that I was unable to stop myself from letting escape... you remember how I mocked one day that poor lover who wept in front of us: eh, well, my friend, I was acting just like him; but it was, in me, the effect of a delicious emotion, and like the emanation of feeling: Adelaïde smiled; I heard Ursule's guarded sighs. What a charming night! it hardly lasted; the hours seemed like minutes, and I had the satisfaction of noticing that Madame Des Tianges and her lovable sister found them no longer than I did. Adelaïde, on our return, assured me that without me, she would not have been at B**'s house in your absence: she spoke to me about those tumultuous gatherings in a tone to persuade me that they are nothing but amusing.

I see Ursule three times a week; and my respect as well as my love do not cease to increase. How many distractions I could have avoided if my good fortune had brought Madame Des Tianges to me sooner! For example, I would not have had on my hands at present that unfortunate intrigue with D***. I had not seen that woman again since the day when, for the first time, Adelaïde brought me to the convent to see her sister. B** informs me this morning that she is furious; I couldn't care less; one must pay no attention to those indecent women, who throw themselves around a man's neck, then drop him with the same impudence: but, if Madame Des Tianges, if my Ursule, should come to find out about that adventure... I would really like to avoid that. For I know D***: if she discovers that I pass the hours at your place now, she will tell the stupidest stories, she will hold the most impertinent discourses... and given it will not be too long before she discovers the truth, after what she saw at the ball, she is the kind of woman to dishonor herself in order to ruin things for me with Adelaïde and Ursule. A Prostitute, a Dancer of the Opera, are less dangerous than those kinds of woman... My God! if my adorable mistress were to think that I had seen D***, since I had sworn to her an undivided and limitless tenderness! My dear Des Tianges, the idea of it makes me shudder; she makes me feel all the value of innocent behavior... I do not suppose that you could do something about it... But no, no; let's wait still; perhaps nothing like what I fear will happen; and I am concerned lest a confidence of the sort would be too disagreeable an indiscretion.

We plan to sup together this even at my uncle's, and Madame Des Tianges is supposed to bring Ursule along with.

I have read your objections, my friend; and as you want me to respond, I will do so voluntarily. You will let me know if my replies are satisfactory. Besides, I believe it is necessary to give an account of the motives for each Article of Rule: that will be the means for preventing objections that others would not fail to make, if this Plan should escape your hands, and to explain some of its Articles which might surprise or revolt readers.

Section IV. Responses to Objections that Each Article of Rule Could Give Rise to

Article 1. It would suffice, in the beginning, to take possession of particular houses that would help to keep expenses down: not all conveniences would be found at first, but one could wait until the Establishment had enough money to fund them; in the meantime, public women collected from every which where would disappear entirely from public view; one would have the advantage of starting the new house with received subjects as prescribed by Article 6 of the Rule: those girls would have, by that means, no commerce with the incorrigible and corrupted poor wretches who have rotted away for so long in the mud.[61] The Parthénions, in addition to the advantages already known, would still have nearly the effect of the *Conservatories* in Italy, which are houses where one receives women and girls whom poverty could drag into debauchery; *vide* the last disposition of *Article 16*.

A fine of *five hundred livres*, or even more, depending on the net worth of the delinquents, that they would incur, all those who in contempt of the law lodged with known public women, is the most effective means that one could employ; above all if one granted the prescribed reward to the informer, and ensured secrecy when he asked for it.

Article 2. I do not believe that one can all of a sudden prohibit kept women as one can prostitutes. That must be delegated to the rank of those whom the good administration of the *Parthénion* will direct; but an active and too prompt execution of which ought to

---

[61]Original footnote: I imagine that in *Paris* the habitable interior of *New-Hall* could at first be employed, to satisfy the particulars, without the least in the world hindering the usage to which that edifice is consecrated for public utility; one would erect double gates on all the streets that lead there; during the day they would all be open, but one would fix an hour in the evening when those gates would be closed, and guarded on the inside by a *Governess*: at the first entry, there would be a small door, through which one would introduce men at the grating to the *Bureau's* loge, situated between the two barriers; there, one would hand over the ticket, and for all the rest, one would follow, as much as possible, the dispositions of the *Rules*. It would be necessary for a second guardroom to be at hand; the one near the Oratory could be moved there. That would be, while waiting for better, an easy way to begin the reform, by forbidding Prostitutes to infect all the quarters of the Capital. (One could even, in London, select one of those vast Buildings that exist in large numbers near *Covent Garden* or *Leicester Field*.)

be regarded as hateful and little practicable; seeing that that would be to submit to an unjust and hard inquisition a number of honest women and girls who would find difficultly in lodging themselves there. One sees that the present system remediates it indirectly by Articles 18, 24, and 29.

Article 3. From the moment one wants to reform, one must employ all means so that the reform is constant and easy to maintain; the shame is in the vice, and not in the precautions one takes against it.

Article 4. This idea is not new: it is what was practiced previously in the principal cities of the Realm. See the first comment in Note L for more on that subject.

As for the Governesses, it is clear that taking into consideration the functions of their positions, their employment cannot be filled except by those whom I have designated.

Article 5. Exercise of the charge of Administrator will be done with order and decency: one would choose only from among too-honest citizens, to govern the *Parthénions*, to administer their revenue, to instill a respectful fear into libertines, founded on wise conduct, exempt of any reproach by the Administrative Members of Council. The disposition of this Article, which forbids them entry into the house, supports Articles 18, 24, 28, 29 and those same Articles make their wisdom felt: those serious men must not however be suspected of loving a *Parthénion* girl. The last measure requests for Administrators the same privilege merely as enjoy companies as little useful as the *Arquebusiers*.

Article 6. What the beginning of this Article prescribes has two motives, both very powerful; the first, to open a safe asylum for girls, which removes them from the temptation of contravening the first Article; the second is to nowise divulge information about their family. The last disposition, which has to do with age, is essential to the proposed Establishment. There could be exceptions however for beauty and talent.

Article 7. The disposition of this one can cause revulsion at first glance; but it is necessary that it be followed to the letter; as much to remove from parents any hope of a useless vengeance, and thereby make them avoid a scene that they themselves will be the first to repent of, as to assure the tranquility of the *Parthénion* subjects. (Those parents will be thus deprived of their natural right over their daughters, to punish them for not having sufficiently looked after their education.)

Article 8. It is absolutely necessary to use a great deal of indulgence in an Establishment such as this one; rigor would render it impracticable; one knows the reason why. *To consider the least evil for a good,* is its motto: this Plan, in itself, is not a good, it is merely the extreme diminutive of an evil incomparably much greater than it appears, and which one cannot imagine.

Article 9. The same motive is at work in this one; if a girl from the *Parthénion* is seen on the gallows, what effect would that not produce, against the proposed goal, which is to attract all those whom a miserable penchant leads into Prostitution and to make them imagine in these houses a more advantageous and gentler fate than they could obtain on their own, or among despicable *madams*, whom the Government is forced to tolerate, despite their crimes? Let no one tell me that I propose a temptation for vice; I appeal to all reasonable individuals; the Establishment that I sketch out will never tempt an honest girl: she will always be sufficiently stopped by the mark of infamy imprinted by our mores and by nature on the last of professions; and for the others, it is better that they come to the *Parthénion* than that they go elsewhere.

Article 10. I repeat; men must be attracted to our Establishment; not to inspire in them a love of debauchery, but to divert them from seeking women whom they would continue to expose themselves to. How many are there today, who, after having lost their health, transmit a shameful malady to their virtuous spouse, and give to the State subjects destined to become useless burdens! I have reason to believe that, by the order prescribed in this Article and the one following it, all will be executed without confusion, and, above all, that scandal will not at all be advertised.

Article 11. This Article tends to the already expressed goal of rendering so easy an access to the Establishment that one does not at all go seeking pleasure elsewhere.

Article 12. One may choose from among a multitude of pretty girls: the girl, in turn, must feel no repugnance for the man who asks for her; one senses just how such a method removes from Prostitution what is most revolting, brutal, and fierce in it.

Article 13. There is nothing here that is not just; we lead back to nature, as much as possible, a condition that falls so far below it: the choice by a man has been free; that by a girl should also be. If the Plan sought merely to provide for physical love, these precautions would be perfectly pointless: far be it from me the thought of having wished to lower man that far; the distinction between the physical and the moral never existed in the thinking man; for him, to love is to enjoy; and to enjoy is to love. One must not imagine that the means proposed for obviating a general refusal might lead to a rather large number of difficulties: as for the rest of it, those cases will be rare, and one could, with certain faces, suddenly employ the proposed means. This Article comes to the aid of 7, whose execution it makes easy: a girl who would have recognized one of her relatives, or friends of the family, will tell her secret to the Governess, so that she might avoid requesting his number.

Articles 14 and 15. These two Articles have for their object the maintenance of order and tranquility, for which there is no such thing as taking too many precautions. They are a follow-up to Articles 10 and 11.

Article 16. This Article's details are necessary, so that everyone might be sure to find at the *Parthénion* what he desires. I sustain even that one must not by any means exclude men of a *certain state*, provided they avoid scandal. How many men have we not seen among those who have imprudently committed themselves to a chimerical perfection, who are carried away by a furious passion, have abused the confidence and secret that certain practices demand, whose utility I do not pretend to attack, in order to instill shame and despair into the heart of the girl's unfortunate parents![62] What terminates this Article puts forth another good that will result from the Establishment: that is, it will keep from disorder a number of young people, and return them to society.

Article 17. It is certain that girls who live in regularity, and who are always clean, will attract instead the type of men for whom I destine the *Outmoded*, rather than those unfortunate, dirty, drunk, corrupt wretches whom they currently associate with. Rates for the first, second, and third Corridors are the most ordinary prices requested by girls who are much beneath those that the proposed Establishment will furnish.[63] The *fourth* is not set too high for men of leisure who love their pleasure, and who often lose their health, paying dearly for it. It will be necessary to set the *fifth* high enough to discourage the masses. As for the *sixth*, it would be more prudent still, to charge *ten louis* instead of *four*.[sic] The rest of this Article prescribes precautions that must be taken in order not to turn away any sums that might be put into the Bureau's coffers, where the tickets are deposited, and shows the wisdom of the disposition of Article 3, which orders capital punishment for any assistant who would let the Receipts be seen. The pur-

---

[62]Original scholium: See *Note N*.

[63]Original footnote: Viz. the current state of Prostitution, *Note A*, towards the end.

pose of the precautions taken in the manner of placing money in the first box is to prevent any difficulties that might arise between men and the Governesses; for in the case where the first might wish to deceive, the Governess will always have before her eyes the legal tender, which she will not drop into the box until after the ticket, and the man has left; if she inserted it into the coffer beforehand, she would be cited, and held responsible for the amount.

Article 18. This will appear perhaps contrary to the goal of the Establishment, and I admit that one would be right in so thinking, if it was not more than probable that the house should always have a sufficient number of Subjects. One could even consider what I propose in this Article as a means to preventing the ruin of families: how many men are pillaged by sirens who make it an honor and a game to deceive them, by despoiling them? Here, that negative consequence will not take place: a lover, in addition to being sure of the faithfulness of his mistress, will be able to rely on the one expense that the house requires: that expense will always be diminishing, in that he will not pay more than 42 livres per week, when his mistress will have exceeded *sixteen years* of age; 33 livres 12 sous when she turns *eighteen*; 25 livres 4 sous, when she will have reached *twenty*; 16 livres 16 sous when the girl is *twenty-five*; 14 livres when she is *thirty*; the price will not go below this, for as long as he keeps his lover. This is also designed to favor titular lovers, whom one has reduced to *twelve livres* per day, the rate for girls in the *sixth*, and to *six livres* for those in the *fifth*, that being the most honest way to proceed, and needs to be encouraged. That which regards children tends as much to the satisfaction of the fathers, as to their discharge from the house. The clauses of the following dispositions are designed to prevent disorders that might result from the freedom men had to go with a girl *kept* by another, and to assure the execution of Article 28.

Article 19. The proposed Establishment must not favor dishonorable unions: looked at from a different angle, it would be unjust to deprive freedom of choice from those who are masters of themselves. I believe however that it would be absolutely necessary to declare as null and void, *by virtue of the law*, any marriage contracted by a man distinguished at birth or by his position, with a girl from the *Parthénion*, if he had happened, by giving a false name, to obtain the Administrative Council's consent; and that, even if the girl had never seen anyone but him. This Article clearly shows the necessity of entrusting the Administration of *Parthénions* only to the most honest of citizens; in other words, to men who add high morals to sufficient intelligence, in order to judge in these important cases.

Article 20. Reason, more than nature, prescribes this conduct: one will give children to their fathers; because by executing my plan, fathers will pay all the expenses, and ought to enjoy all the advantages.

Article 21. There is no disadvantage to according these prerogatives to fathers, titular lovers. But this Article has other dispositions that will not appear clear: one may ask, for example, what was I trying to say by having these fathers who, being unable to contract marriage, leave half their property? I reply only that the abuses that reign are infinitely more dangerous than what I would occasion, which, in itself, has nothing that shocks nature, nor reason even or ancient Laws.[64] Of course, those fathers will avoid scandal, which must always be punished in a well-run State.

Articles 22 and 23. These two Articles decide how all hours of the day are to be employed. An Establishment without rule falls into a kind of anarchy, which destroys the utility that one proposes to draw from it. One will teach the girls all that might contribute to making them amiable: so that nobody might be scandalized, I will make the motive known: Article 8 of that section.

Article 24. This tends again to relieve the house, and to give to men a certain freedom, which makes them prefer coming to the Establishment, compared to all other means of procuring a mistress. (It is

---

[64]Original footnote: The Council of Trent raised the question whether Priests could marry. It was decided in the negative, for reasons that appeared good apparently; for this being merely a point of discipline, the holy Synod decided based on human motives, with the aid of merely natural insight. Consequently, it could have been mistaken: it is the sentiment of all Theologians. I have read somewhere that Erasmus, the famous Erasmus, speaking of the Ecclesiastics and Monks of his time who were married, instead of treating with decency so important a point of Morality, was amused to joke about it like a schoolboy. "*At ista omnis tragœdia,*" he said, "*exit in catastrophen comicam. Uhi contigit uxo, occinitur: Valete & plaudite.*"

A man, whose virtue, good behavior, and intelligence nobody would contest, the Abbot Saint Peter, strongly influenced by Nature's obligations, had consecrated one day a week to propagation. *Dictionary of Encyclopedia*, under the word "Population."

good to observe that the freedom that kept girls enjoy by having a titular lover, the presents they might receive, will make them desirous to assume that role, and that those reasons will prevent them from refusing a man who otherwise would not be to their liking.)

Article 25. On freedom. It is rather enough not to be able to leave the house without adding still more weight to their chains within it. And to oblige them, in an effective manner, to enjoy the permitted amusements that are procured for them, everything that could distract their attention will be suppressed. They will not be ordered to read, to work, but the alternative is to do suchlike or be bored.

Articles 26 and 27. Many reasons have determined me to propose *Article 26*: the girls who are the object of it are returned from a tryst, and it is presupposed that they will not lapse into excess; they are small enough in number, in limited proportion to the men who may lay claim to them only; those men moreover have less fantasies, are more easily satisfied than those of a more acute condition: the *Outmoded* women would be too dependent on the house if things were otherwise; but that reason would be worthless if the first did not exist. Those who will have appeared one or two times on the same day can ask to leave the communal hall for the rest of the time. They will be watched closely, and the Head Governess will pay the most scrupulous attention to the health of those girls.

Article 28. The severity of this Article will infuse a kind of chastity into the very heart of Prostitution. Impudicity is an abuse of the act of procreation, and nothing is more contrary to the propagation of the species. That is why ancient Moralists recommended purity. The most virtuous men were chaste; it remains to be seen whether absolute continence is not criminal. One could respond that the example risks so little danger of it, and that the effect it produces on others is always excellent; the total abstinence of women is not detrimental, or, if one wishes, *culpable*, except in the individual who has turned it into a law; on the other hand, incontinence publicly displayed by men and women would have frightening effects, would spill over onto everything, even preference, and would turn love into a cause without effect. But the effect of love is the procreation of humans.

Article 29. All this would be necessary, and ought to be practiced to the letter: the Administrative Council will be unable to budge from it.

Article 30. The amount being fixed, for clothing, for the entire year, by the Accounts *Payable* and *Receivable*,[65] it is natural that each girl shall be free to chose the stuff, and the means of employing it, which adorns her the most advantageously. Girls destined for marriage, or to become mothers, and the Laborers raised in the house, which *Article 38* speaks to, could be dressed in the old clothes discarded by Subjects of the *Parthénion*; those habits being still very proper, given the care that the Governesses will oblige the girls to take with them.

Article 31. Baths are not, since the usage of linen is so widespread, as frequent among us as they

---

[65]Original footnote: See *that Accounting*, Letter XI, section V.

ought to be: it is certain that a warm bath encourages the *transudation* of an enormous amount of impurities, which cause regrettable deposits, and often mortal maladies, above all to sedentary people: another advantage of a bath for women is a lightening of the complexion of those who are too dark.[66]

Article 32. Cosmetics, in general, do more ill than good, particularly for pretty girls: they wrinkle their visages, gnaw at their natural colors, and hasten the appearance of decrepitude. (The preceding Article counsels a thing nearly out of fashion; the present one forbids doing oneself up; the omission of a bath is unreasonable, and the practice of makeup pernicious; let us reestablish good habits, and suppress bad ones.)

Article 33. A bevy of miserable souls, lodged on the outskirts of the faubourgs, arrive each evening in the center of town to communicate their corruption to useful and strong men, whose lack of fortune has turned them into servants of humanity; men of a sort, I cannot prevent myself from saying it, of an entirely different worth, for society in general, than the most enlightened Author,[67] than the idling Bourgeois, the cunning Merchant, the impertinent Shop Assistant,

---

[66]Original footnote: "the skin's grime, retained in the pores, or on the superficies, is capable of producing numerous maladies, like boils, phlegmons, &c.; scabies and dry patches are principally engendered by that grime; one must obviate these maladies, precisely by washing the skin through baths, frictions, and other means appropriate to lift the grime from the body's circumference. The inhabitants of warm climates, who are more subject to grime on the skin, because of the heat of the climate where they live, bathe quite often, to heal themselves of those maladies, a method they have retained from the ancients." – *Encyclop.*

and the useless Valet; they are the ones who build our homes, cultivate our gardens, carry our burdens, &c.; must one abandon them inhumanely at the risk of exposing them to a passion that triumphs over the wisest? The abuse that reigns today is greater doubtless than that which *Columelle* takes up, when he says, *this would be to inflict great harm, to give to Workers who are occupied with the most necessary of tasks the means and the facility to see women of pleasure.*[68] That maxim, full of wisdom and reason, will not be elucidated at all: the Rule has provided for it. The manual laborer will not be exposed, nor in his health, nor by the waste of his time, nor in debauchery: I repeat: it is not libertinage that I want to favor: I would despise myself if I had had that thought; it is the consequences of an abuse that has become necessary, that I wish to prevent; it is the evil that I strive to diminish; a cruel illness that I seek to extirpate.

VENEREAL DISEASES

Article 34. This one here is the principal goal of the Establishment: a man will not be allowed to choose a girl, if one is not sure that he is healthy.

Article 35. It is natural that the first duties of the Head Governess should be to ensure exact adherence to the preceding Article, and execution of the following two.

---

[67]Original footnote: "Necessity is above utility: it proceeds at the same pace as the just, the honest, and the holy."

[68]Original footnote: *Quippe plurimum offert mali, si Operario meretricandi potestas fiat.* Columelle. Book II, chapter I.

Article 36. One believes that one owes no consideration to contemptible souls who, knowing themselves to be infected with venereal disease, are so unjust as to want to communicate it to others, and as inimical to themselves as to aggravate their difficulties instead of seeking to find themselves a cure.

Article 37. The attention that one will give to girls suffering from a disease is a necessary consequence of the Establishment, and the most dignant object of the Head Governess' attentions, as well as those who are subordinate to her: the Administration will obtain an exact account of the treatments, and it will promptly remediate any abuses, and above all any negligences, that were introduced. It is in this way that routine and inattention may be avoided. As for the rest of it, all the Articles are so interconnected that lack of observation of a single one of them would soon lead to a violation of all the others.

FATE OF CHILDREN BORN IN THE HOUSE

Article 38. Men are the riches of the State; it is in multiplying them that a Prince increases his power. What joy for the countrysides into which the Militia each year carries a new scare, to see oneself saved by our Establishment![69] The advantage that would result for the State would be immense: there would be several thousands of men who would remain on the land, cultivating the earth: because, for the majority of men

[69]Original footnote: A custom introduced several years earlier, to give *Foundlings* to Laborers, in order to habituate them to work, and to *draft* them into the Militia instead of children from home is a step in the direction that I propose.

who have once quit it, they never return to it at the end of their service; they either become idlers, vagabonds, or at the very least extremely debauched; others, who, without the Militia, *would tend to* the plough or *cultivate* vineyards, grow accustomed to the city, whose soft life enervates them; and those are men for the most part lost to the State.

It is necessary to acknowledge that the male Subjects furnished by the *Parthénions* of the Realm would not by themselves suffice to achieve that goal: but this is only an indication of the means, and not a law; that one might augment that number by Foundlings, who otherwise wither away in the *Pitié-Salpêtrière* and elsewhere; by those in hospitals of the provinces, who spend their youth carding wool, – I believe that one will then have sufficient numbers of them to execute the proposed service. I put forward that those young men will make excellent Soldiers, because since childhood they are raised in submission and in dependence that is as absolute as it is blind for a stranger; they have no relatives at all nor connections; their father is the State; their fatherland, the Realm; they would remain in service for as long as their strength permits it. Those old Soldiers would be employed on difficult occasions, when experience or intrepidness in the face of danger are necessary. One could object that those troops will be vilified by others. May God forfend that I should look on the state of the Military of France or England as so poorly disciplined as to insult, with gladness in my heart, a body of brave fellows by making a crime out of their birth, which was not their doing.

The second disposition has to do with the girls: one will benefit from those who are disgraced by nature, by employing them usefully around the house; others will choose the state they want to embrace. One could say that the dowry I propose to assign to them is considerable, given their large numbers. I respond that girls with a pretty face will compose the tenth part of the children, and I believe that the *Parthénion*, well managed, well administered, can suffice for that expense; it is something that I plan to prove at a later time.[70] One might still object that the house has quite a few expenses: the *Outmoded*, the girls who are ill, the costly manner in which I propose to maintain the Subjects of the house on every point, &c. I acknowledge the justice of those remarks; but a means for helping the house would naturally present itself, if it should be that it had need of assistance: the *Salpêtrière Hospital;* becomes almost unnecessary; one could place elsewhere the insane who might be locked up there, and one would allocate to our Establishment the revenues of that house. I will go even further; I dare maintain that the Hospitals do not fulfill, by large measure, the goal of utility that their Founders had envisioned, and do not procure the relief that the poor are believed to receive from them; half the Realm does not have them, and are all the better for it. Let's leave Hôtel-Dieu alone, while we're at it; in a city like Paris, it is absolutely necessary that there be a place where the indigent might die as they lived,[71] in the bosom of horror, and in the arms of despair... O! sad humanity! where are your acorns and your forests!... All other Hospitals are

---

[70]Original footnote: *See* Letter XI.

harmful, support idleness, and deceive the ill finally, who have imprudently relied on those Establishments, and which have not done a thing for them over the course of a lifetime. They hope to find tranquility there, and repose; they meet with nothing but an early hell: I say this, because I have seen it; death is a lesser evil than the sad life one leads in our Hospitals;[72] to suppress them, or redirect all their revenue to a house fo r *pregnant girls, Foundlings,* and our *Establishment,* that would be merely to destroy one evil in order to make a greater good. But what will become of those poor souls whose benefit is so meager a thing, which barely gives them their daily bread? If this were the place, I would respond... Des Tianges, those immense goods that people with soft hands possess, why were they given to them? doubtless to nourish our Prelates and our Abbesses in a luxurious indolence; in a soft idleness, that useless Carthusian monk, that sensual Bernardin, &c. A swarm of locusts has landed on the property of the poor and devours it, and one is surprised that they die of hunger! If this wasn't the place, I would say that we other Financiers should turn our parks into arable fields... but I will be quiet: I add only this, that next winter I am going to tear up the flowerbeds at ***, my broad sand-strewn

---

[71]Original footnote: In other words: *Where they die promptly*: one has, in that house (and in another), a very particular care not to let the sick, and above all the aged, languish.

[72]Our Hospitals: for comparison purposes, the curious reader should see Paul Verlaine's autobiographical essay, *Mes Hôpitals*, which treats of the author's experiences in French hospitals of the mid to late 19th century (one hundred years after this work) during the course of his, mostly later, life, and published in 1891. See *My Hospitals and My Prisons*, Sunny Lou Publishing, 2020.

paths, and I am going to dedicate nearly one league of expensively unproductive land to agriculture.

As for the manner of dressing people of the house, I believe that nothing particular is needed: decency itself is absolutely demanded. He who said that the divers *estates* ought to be marked by different styles of dress had not thought his idea through deeply enough certainly. That distinction among men is hateful, principally in our mores: it would tend merely to nourish the impertinent vanity of a small number of men, while covering in confusion (displaced, to be honest, but not the less painful) the *third-estate* almost entirely, which is a thousand times more numerous than the other two combined; it would thus satisfy the pleasure of one man at the expense of nine hundred ninety-nine others: never has such a Law been proposed, unless it were in Morocco, or, if one likes, in the unfortunate Empire of the Incas, since the time that Europeans unjustly conquered it.[73]

Article 39. The disposition of that Article will retain the *Parthéniens* in their duty. It would be hoped that the punishment for seducers was widespread. In a country where Laws and Religion prevent divorce, one needs extraordinary remedies: I know no one more criminal or more contemptible than a woman who deceives her husband, unless it be her seducer.[74]

Article 40. The hope of becoming a Governess, or at least to teach one day the Arts to the

---

[73]never has such a Law...: in fact, the Chinese had, prior to the Chinese Revolution, precisely such laws, going back at least as far as the Tang Dynasty. Editor's note.

girls, will give some pleasure to the exercises: that re-sort will be less efficacious perhaps for containing the Subjects, than punishments; but also, it has no down-side.

Article 41. It is important not to frighten the girls by the prospect of a painful future.

Article 42. The girls, once admitted into the house, must never leave it. One will no longer meet a prostitute on the street then; by consequence, honest women will never be mistaken for such, and insulted, as they are not sure to be avenged immediately. The scandal that Prostitutes give rise to, by showing them-selves, will be removed. Another advantage is that, without the bait presented to them by the girls they encounter, and who awaken in them their calmed de-sires, men would often avoid the crime. Nor will one be anxious for the inconveniences so greatly to be feared, if Prostitution were suppressed, of debauchees not finding any way to release their penchants: they will have in the *Parthénions* an ever-ready resource.

[74]Original footnote: *Parthéniens*, in other words, the children of prostitutes. In Sparta, there were young people who bore that name; here's their story. Lacedaemonia was waging a stubborn war with the Messenians for several years. The Spartans, assuming that it would be a long one, were afraid lest the distance they had put between themselves and their wives would prejudice the Republic, by exposing it to a lack of new Citizens: they sent to Sparta unmarried young men, and ordered them to have, indiscriminately, traffic with all the girls. That commission was duly executed, such that twenty years later Lacedaemonia found itself in the necessity of expulsing all the children that resulted from it; because being in great number and not having any inheritance to hope for, they were a drag on the Republic. They called them the *Parthéniens*, from the Greek root Παρθέν, girl, due to their knowing only who their mother was, who had given birth to them.

This Article exempts, from the rule that it establishes, anyone who becomes married, and who, having become mistress of herself, due to the death of her parents, and become heir to a property sufficient to live on, would like to go out and govern it. That is nothing but just and reasonable. The power that the house will hold over them is necessary for containing them, or making disorders cease, as our Establishment ought to prevent everything.

Article 43. This Article shows in what spirit the Administrators must govern the house, and the necessity of assigning that position only to virtuous Citizens: in every way, the honest man almost always does good, and the scoundrel bad.

Article 44. *Two evils to avoid a worse one*. Do not listen to fanatics: those sorts of people talk a lot; they cry out loudly and never reflect. In London, where the Theaters are closed on Sundays, one gets drunk, one gambles, and one goes to visit *women of pleasure*. It would be much better to open the Theaters, and watch a play by *Shakespeare* or *Dryden*; it would be more decent, doubtless, to watch *Cato* by *Addison*, than to stagnate in a tavern, or not to leave it except by going to fisticuffs.

Article 45. A house in the Country that has too many Subjects must send them to the Capital, and thus for all the rest, without any particular Administration being able to refuse: one could similarly exchange Subjects received in a Provincial town, or in the Capital, with other Subjects, in order to distance girls from their acquaintances; and that would become even absolutely necessary in the Countryside.

The Capital, lacking Subjects, will draw from *Parthénions* in the Countryside, as much as is needed. It is understood why it must enjoy that privilege.

(A certain number of men in the Capital, much more vile than Prostitutes, will lose to the new Establishment their means of livelihood. Those despicable men are ordinarily the authors of many secret murders. They pass their lives in a villainous idleness founded on greed: all their talent resides in insulting, in fighting then, they are cowardly and like assassins. They have a name, which was formerly considered a disgrace: Machærophorus[75], which signifies none other than *Gendarme*: but that word, from which one has dropped the last two syllables, is quite vile ever since it characterizes[76] them.)

I don't know if I have attained my goal, by proposing the 45 Articles of the Rule that I have sent to you, my dear friend, and whether I have forgotten anything essential. *It belongs to men only, who have merited some distinction in their handling of business affairs, to weigh in* on this important subject; and I would respectfully wait for their decision before I made it public. I have tried not to lose sight of that wise maxim: *The power of Laws will only regulate the passions, not destroy them.* You will determine

____

[75]Original scholium: Μαχαεροφόρος, swordsman.

[76]Original footnote: Here is the etymology of that villainous term: *Maqu...* The *Encyclopedic Dictionary* gives to the word *Put...* an Italian origin, and derives *Putana* from it: one could also say that it comes from the Spanish *Puta*: in truth, neither language gave it to us: it comes from the French *Pute*, which one pronounces still as "poot" or "peut, "peute," in diverse provinces; an expression formed by the Latin *Putidus, puant, puante* [stinking].

from where you sit whether I have satisfied every reasonable objection that one could make... It is eight o'clock, I fly to your house to pay a visit: bye for now.

* * *

Good day, my good friend, – I say good day because my watch shows three o'clock in the morning. I escorted your spouse and her sister home from my uncle's house at one o'clock; we had a small chat, as you can see. However, I come back to you, and I want to end my Letter before going to bed.

Never has a boisterous party satisfied me like that tranquil, even serious, supper at a respectable Old Man's place, surrounded by sensible family members. Joy broke out sometimes, but it was the laughter of reason. As for my uncle, he was in a particularly charming mood. I don't know if he noticed my passion for Ursule; it seemed to me that his cheerfulness was redoubled when he saw the looks, the attention, I paid to that lovely girl. He addressed her a word, from time to time, and it was always to pay her some compliment. I cannot express to you how happy his remarks made me; for, my dear friend, although I might be rich, and my own master, I feel, ever since I have started loving Ursule, my feelings for my relatives to increase, and I am delighted to do nothing that would displease them. Starting tomorrow, I want to open my heart to them. I will wait for your return, to introduce to you what he said to me.

I embrace you a thousand times, dear Des Tianges; my friendship for you is so great that I do not think that the kind, the tender, Adelaïde is more attached to you than is

   – D'ALZAN.

Ninth Letter

From the Same.

June 9, 176*.

Yesterday morning, I went to my uncle's, whom I did not find the day before; I was received by him with demonstrations of the greatest friendship. After we had chatted some time about the current events, and other indifferent things, I was about to speak with him about the reason for my visit: he had anticipated me.

"You are twenty-five years old, nephew," he said to me. "It is time you made a choice. At your age, one is no longer a novice; you know the world, the mistakes one must avoid, as well as the social virtues necessary to be acquired: you are not, I hope, so foolish as to let yourself be taken in solely by two beautiful eyes, and I believe you are too reasonable not to seek more solid advantages in the object of your choice."

That preamble caught me off guard, and I wanted to interrupt him: but he gestured to me to let him finish.

"When a person gets married, it is a durable engagement that one contracts, and it does not resemble those little flings that you have had everywhere." (He gave me a long list of my known mistresses, and, to my great astonishment, he finished with D***.) "An honest man must love his wife, and her alone. I have my eye on you, my dear D'Alzan: but I would first like to be sure that you have for the woman I destine for you the feelings she is worthy to inspire. She is beautiful, rich, and above all that, virtuous, modest, reasonable. I knew her mother. I was in love with her when we were both young and free: another man got the upperhand on me; he knew how to please her more. I was devastated; but finally, I was upset only with myself; and I renounced from that moment forward seeking a relationship with anyone else, which could not be happy. My esteem and my respect for that lovely woman did not at all diminish; but I went to great effort to avoid seeing her again. She became a widow eventually: when her mourning had passed, when I believed her tears were dry, I was going to offer her my hand, and to entreat her to allow me to serve as a father to her children. Her death, several years ago, removed that sweet hope. Judge for yourself if that was not a serious blow for me. She left two girls, rich, and under a wise Tutor. Watching them grow, I thought of you. The oldest one in particular, who just married one of our own, would have really suited you; but her marriage was arranged so promptly that I was not made aware of it until things had gotten too far along. With God's grace, the younger sister is not inferior to the older, not in merit, not in beauty, and I have wanted to act promptly in order not to be caught off guard a second time. I spent all day yesterday with Monsieur *Laurens*, my friend, godparent of the older sister, and tutor to them both; I made him acquainted with my idea; we took off together immediately for the young person's Convent. Monsieur *Laurens* explained to her the purpose of our visit, and when I mentioned my nephew's name, that dear girl blushed prodigiously; she was, at that moment, more beautiful than an angel; I could not help from crying out loud, '*My, how that rascal D'Alzan is a lucky man!*' The young demoiselle did not give us a positive answer, but (and note this) she referred us to her *dear sister*, whose orders she said she followed to the letter. From the air of satisfaction that dominated her visage, we could tell that our proposition did not displease her. We went today to visit her sister..."

"Pardon me, my dear uncle," I interrupted him, "but all this is rather pointless, I believe; I am desperate to tell you that your views do not coincide with my own: I am in love, if that word can express all that a young woman inspires in me, with whom all that you have said just now perfectly accords, but it is not she. My dear uncle, I repeat, or rather, my father, as you deign to stand in for him for so long, my pain is extreme, being unable to demonstrate to you on this occasion my deference to your least desires; but you will not be inexorable, for you too have loved."

"It would not happen to be D***," my uncle retorted testily, "that makes you speak in this way? If I had thought... My dear child, for God's sake, you must realize that you could not love that contemptible woman for more than one week, even if you had the most tenacious constancy..."

"You wrong me, Monsieur," I replied, "I am not seeing D***; I no longer see her at all, since I have met the touching object that charms me."

"In that case... you are right: what I have just told you could not possibly fit Madame D***. I would have thought that the woman I propose..."

"Uncle, she may be charming, but I am under the spell of another, as I have told you."

"'She *may be charming!'* Honestly, D'Alzan, you are incomprehensible. Always fussing over women whom you lavish with incense and adulations, whom you badmouth no sooner than you leave them. How could they not deceive you, those whose vanity makes them credulous? I deceive myself sometimes even, when I look at you. For example, the other day, you visited me, with that young person whom I have just spoken to you about, I could have sworn that you were in love with her; and I said as much to Madame Des Tianges, her sister, even..."

"Wait...what did you just say? Madame Des Tianges! The woman you give to me is the sister of Madame Des Tianges!"

"Yes, what do you find so surprising, so marvelous, about that... But what do all these transports mean?" (I was on my knees at this point, my good friend.)

"Ah! Monsieur," I exclaimed, "she is the one I love."

Imagine for yourself, my friend, all the different phases that I passed through successively; my trances, my alarms, and the joy that I felt suddenly. The cause of my error was the name *Laurens,* which my uncle attributed to your father, which name nobody knows him by, and which you have never mentioned to me. Monsieur *De Longepierre's* satisfaction was as real and almost as great as my own. He demonstrated as much to me in a thousand ways; he wants to assure me that everything in his possession will be mine after his death, and that he plans, from this moment forward, to make a considerable gift to me; he calls Ursule his daughter; our union will reacquire for him the happiness he was deprived of.

We agreed that I would pay a visit to Madame Des Tianges, to let her know that Monsieur *De Longepierre* would be paying her a visit; after I reflected that it was still too early, I went home again; and I write to you while waiting for the moment to go and share the good news with my best friend. I believe her already instructed as to the steps that my uncle has made, yesterday, regarding Ursule with your father... My friend, how my heart beats! It seems to me that I am about to inform Madame Des Tianges that I love Ursule... As to what I feel right now, one could say I am afraid... Delightful timidity!... it proves to me, my dear friend, that I love Mademoiselle *De Roselle* as she deserves to be loved. Time drags on: my watch is slow I think... I leave you...

Ah! Des Tianges! Des Tianges!... look... a note!... it is from your wife!

NOTE
From Madame Des Tianges to D'Alzan

You are for me, Monsieur, an indefinable person: you have taken a brilliant step forward with respect to Ursule, through your uncle and your friend's father;

*you prove to me the tenderest feelings that you have for my sister; and all that at the same time that a criminal and dishonorable intrigue binds you to... how shall I say it, Monsieur? to D***; a whore, who would be offended if one doubted it. Ah, D'Alzan! Adelaïde would not have believed you to be two-faced, a villain, a seducer: she supposed you only weak, light, ruined by the century... Ingrate! was it necessary to choose the sister of Monsieur Des Tianges, your friend, for the unfortunate victim of your hypocrisy! Poor Ursule!... you do not deserve the tears she will shed... Listen to me, you who are the cause of them; you, who betrayed my confidence and my friendship, and that of my husband, which are the most sacred things among men, given that you have abused our love; never show your face again before Ursule or me; grant me that favor, I request it; and if that does not suffice, I forbid it... forever.*

— ADELAÏDE DES TIANGES

My good, dear friend!... I will die before you arrive... Ursule will think me false, vile... My past behavior will not reassure her... Des Tianges! I would give my blood... But... oh! that idea slays me... One moment... that Ursule should think me for one moment... Write to them... hurry up and write to them, and justify me in their eyes... I am innocent, you know it; but they will refuse to hear me out... Madame Des Tianges... Ah! it is her virtue... friendship.... that she believes is betrayed... which will block me... remove to me all access... Ursule... My friend, I am gripped... My hand, all my body, so violent a trembling seizes me... I cannot write any more... Adieu... adieu, my dear friend.

    – D'Alzan

Tenth Letter

From Monsieur D'Alzan de Longepierre to
Des Tianges.

Same day, evening.

I write to you in haste, Monsieur, very sad, very afflicted; your family and mine are standing around the bed of Monsieur D'Alzan, your friend, my poor nephew. He finds himself poorly, this morning, at ten o'clock. You know that impudent Madame D***; it is her fault, it is her perfidy that has reduced him to the state he is in.

It is not two hours earlier that he left my home: we had agreed to meet at your place. I went there; I was surprised not to see him, and even more surprised by the coldness with which Madame Des Tianges received me, whom I thought he had instructed as to our conversation from earlier. I ask for him, after initial compliments. Your wife responded to me that she believes Monsieur D'Alzan ought not to return to her house. I stood confused: I pressured Madame Des Tianges to tell me more. She begged me to spare her, and sent me to see my nephew, who would inform me, she added, much better than she could do. Already troubled by so unexpected an event, I flew to your friend's house, and I find him... alas! I haven't the strength to pronounce the word: the state in which I found him, it seized me. He returned home, and Madame Des Tianges' door had just been shut on him: the distraction of his reason was painted in his look... He did not recognize me, he did not see me! add to that a burning fever, sobs, long sighs; that is a picture of the situation. I myself helped carry him to his bed. At the end of several moments, he recognized me; he pressed my hand, but he did not say anything yet; I saw in his eyes that he was looking for something; I saw where he was looking; noticing a Letter open on his bureau, which he seemed to stare at, I took it up: it informed me only too well. I asked my poor ill man whether it was not what had put him into so violent a state? He made a sign to me: yes. I assured him that I could justify him in the minds of Madame Des Tianges and her sister. That promise made an impression on him. He spoke to me:

"Ah! run then, my dear uncle," he said to me, in a feeble voice, "and give me my life back, if there is still time; it is absolutely necessary that I see them again, that I speak with them, and that will I die if I cannot persuade them of my innocence."

I did not waste a single moment. On returning to your house, I surprised Madame Des Tianges by my strange plea: "Save my nephew, madame," I cried out to her; "your note has put him in a state that will frighten you: bring Mademoiselle De Roselle with you; he wants to speak with you both, to destroy the calumnies that have blackened his name, or to die: I will answer for his innocence; you have been deceived: come, I entreat you; I will set you straight on all that..." I expressed myself with such vehemence that I had not noticed the impression my discourse was making on the dear Madame Des Tianges: she looked pale and was trembling.

"Oh, Sir! what has happened then?" she said to me. "Let's go, Monsieur, let's leave; we will go wherever you wish us to. Let's climb into your carriage and pick my sister up along the way."

Along the way, she overwhelmed me with questions; I satisfied her to the best of my abilities; as regards the trouble that I found myself in. She spoke to me of D***; she told me that that woman had come in person to find her; that to add some credence to what she had advanced, she had shown to her notes written by my nephew, the last of which, conceived in very clear terms, was dated the day before. I assured her that the date had been altered, or that the note itself was entirely fabricated. I recounted to her what had happened between D'Alzan and myself that same morning. Whereupon we arrived at the Mademoiselle De Roselle's Convent. Madame Des Tianges filled her in a bit. In my very adversity, I felt a feeling of joy; for I thought I perceived that my nephew did not love an ingrate.

When we appeared in D'Alzan's room, he asked that we be left alone with him... I cannot recall what happened then, without shedding some tears... My nephew justified himself completely... Monsieur Des Tianges' dear wife and the beautiful Ursule stopped at nothing to console him... How touched I was! when I thought... If my dear D'Alzan recovers (for I cannot conceal from you that the Doctors do not dare yet answer for him): if he recovers, I say, as I hope, by the tender attentions and kindnesses of the two sisters, he will look upon that accident as a stroke of good luck. He wanted to exonerate himself entirely, though Mademoiselle De Roselle and Madame Des Tianges herself exempted him from that charge: he displayed the Letter that D*** wrote to him in response to his note, and the date precedes by nearly a month your departure for Poitiers.

My nephew's domestics have sent an alert to all our family; family members run to him from every quarter. What good is such zeal? all the visitors that D'Azlan desired were reduced to two: the others are uncomfortable, and I am going to free him of them...

– 10 o'clock in the evening.

I have just returned from seeing my nephew; everyone has departed, with the exception of those who have given him his life back. When they appeared to be going away, the convulsions that had seized him in the morning returned with a violence. The two lovely sisters sat down on either side of his bed; the joy that their dear presence brought him calmed his overwrought nerves; he just nodded off, and the Doctors answer for him. On the first assurance that they gave, Madame Des Tianges briskly removed a diamond from her finger, and made him who had just spoken accept it from her. Judge for yourself how much pleasure that small show of affection caused me. That will be the first thing that D'Alzan will hear of when he recovers. I find myself quite well consoled, monsieur, to have something better to announce to you on finishing. I am very perfectly, &c.

– DES TIANGES DE LONGEPIERRE

Eleventh Letter

From D'Alzan to Des Tianges.

June 13.

We receive your letter presently, my good friend, and I obtain permission from Madame Des Tianges to respond myself. That will convince you better than any other thing, of the efficacy of her efforts, and those of my beautiful, my tender, my adorable bride... No, dear brother, from now on nothing can separate D'Alzan from that Ursule whom he adores: yesterday morning, we pronounced the sacred oath that binds us forever each to each. I was doing much better; one could have waited for you; my uncle, your parents, and mine were of one mind; but Adelaïde wanted us to be united in my chamber. What generosity! and how dear was the hand that I received from her! All my life, I will look on Madame Des Tianges as an inestimable friend, like a tender sister, an adored mother, my tutelary divinity. And my bride? Ah! Des Tianges! my heart swims in an ocean of voluptuousness. O what happiness it was to lie next to her, on that alabaster bosom, which you protected while waiting for me. Now that we are married, everything turns for the better. I am considered ill still; and yet, I feel that I have never felt better in my life. I have desired, with all the ardor I am capable of, the hand of Mademoiselle De Roselle: now that I have obtained it, I feel the happiness that I desired even more vividly. It is, my good friend, as if I had not known all the merit, the full value, of the woman I idolized. O women! enchantresses, you clearly hold the middle ground between divinity and man! whoever did not know how to please you, whoever has not been loved by you, has not lived: he has vegetated; but life, the sweet warmth of life, never, never has he felt it. How does it happen that there are men who fear the delicious union of two souls bound tightly together by the same affections, the same goods, by those innocent beings who owe them their life, in a word, by the most sacred Laws of society! If they could form an idea of what I am feeling now... of what we both feel, dear Des Tianges, they would immediately renounce the error that makes them miserable.

This Letter would no longer find you in Poitiers, I addressed it to the Post Master of *Blois*. Your obliging impatience has given us all the greatest pleasure. It is really quite flattering, for your spouse and your friend, to learn, that *you cannot wait* a day, *not a single day without being informed of their situation*. She is happy, dear Des Tianges: you will not find here, on your arrival, anything but signs of the most vivid joy: come, your wife...

From Madame DES TIANGES

...has never desired you more, my dear husband. Come and compensate me for all the trouble your friend has caused me. He is happy, at present: but if you had seen him... He is a child, and I forgive him for everything. I had only one person to console; my sister also was despairing, although she hid it. They have both caused me a great deal of trouble, and I so love them, just as before, with all my heart. Adieu, my friend. If I had the fate of this Letter, I would be embracing you one day earlier.

— ADELAÏDE DES TIANGES

From Madame D'ALZAN

I will come straight to the point, cherished brother, in order to justify the crimes that my sister accuses me of. *I caused her some trouble!* me! she may write that to you! eh, well, she is deceiving you, believe you me. One never causes sorrow, I think, in those whom one loves, unless it is despite oneself; and for that, one must pardon them. No, I could not support the idea of having caused, for one instant, trouble for my adorable sister. My dear Adelaïde gives back to me everything I lost, when heaven took our parents from us. *To have afflicted her!* ah, never, I have never wanted it. What would that mean if I told you... She forbids me to write to you; she does not want me to say it... Eh, well, I will be quiet...

I am quite happy with someone whom you love: someone who has for me and my sister the feelings that I desired: the gift of all my heart, of all my feelings, is the price for it. Nobody after my sister... She no longer looks after me: know that it is I who console her: she could not forgive herself... She returns... Nobody, after my sister, is so sincerely attached to you as

— URSULE D'ALZAN.

From D'Alzan

They took away the quill, my dear friend; we dispute amongst ourselves the pleasure of chatting with you. This Letter will be all the more agreeable to you, as you come to see herein the cherished characters of her who makes you the most fortunate of husbands. In order to prove to you that I carry myself as well as I can, after a rather violent commotion, I want to profit from the moment when a visit obliges them to leave me alone, in order to finish my Plan. You will be amused to verify my calculations in your post chaise: also, I suspect that you will be unable, once you have returned, to find a moment to do so.

Section V. Compensation from the Production of Different Classes, with the Expenses of the Parthénions

It appears rather probable that the number of girls, *Public* and *Kept,* can climb in the Realm to 30,000: 20,000 in the Capital, and 10,000 in the provinces; but I will not base my Establishment on so considerable a number. Let us only suppose that there are, in the city of Paris, *twelve thousand girls, Public* and *Kept*; nearly half in the rest of the Realm. Despite the well-being that the proposed Establishment will procure for *Parthéniennes*, I do not doubt that the prohibition to leave the house and the powerlessness in which the girls will find themselves, to free themselves from profligates who are the fatal accompaniments of Prostitution, will reduce the number of those unfortunate beings; I would subtract another 1,000 even to put things at the lowest level; we shall have then, in the entire Realm, *seventeen thousand girls*, who can be placed in the *Parthénions.*

It is proven by new *Research on the Population* by Monsieur Messence,[77] that nearly one third of men live to *forty-five years of age*. That general rule ought to be double proportionately[78] for prostitutes. Thus, when one has made a choice between the two classes of the *Outmoded*, as Article XXXIII prescribes, there will be at most one thousand girls in all the Realm, at the Establishment's expense. And we will have those who, each day, produce revenue, which exceeds their expenses more or less:

Outmoded... at 6 sous, 500 (400 employed) a day, 120 livres.

Outmoded... at 12 sous, 730 (600 employed)... 360 livres.

First Corridor:

at 18 sous, no. 2, 3000 (2000 employed)... 2,100 livres.

at 1 livre, 4 sous, no. 1, 3000 (2000 employed) ... 2,100 livres.

---

[77]Original footnote: Paris, in-quarto. Durand Nephew, rue Saint-Jacques.

[78]Double proportionately: two thirds will live to 45, presumably.

Second Corridor:

at 1 livre 16 sous, no. 2, 3900 (2000 employed)... 4,200 livres.

at 2 livres, 8 sous, no. 1, 3900 (2000 employed)... 4,200 livres.

Third Corridor:

at 3 livres, no. 2, 4000 (2000 employed)... 6,600 livres.

at 3 livres, 12 sous, no. 1, 4000 (2000 employed)... 6,600 livres.

Fourth Corridor:

at 4 livres 16 sous, no. 2, 3000 (1500 employed)... 8,100 livres.

at 6 livres, no. 1, 3000 (1500 employed)... 8,100 livres.

Fifth Corridor:

at 12 livres, no. 2, 1700 (1000 employed)... 18,000 livres.

at 24 livres, no. 1, 1700 (1000 employed)... 18,000 livres.

Sixth Corridor:

at 96 livres... 170 (85 employed).., 8,160 livres.

Total... (per day)... 9,585... 46,640 livres

(per year)... 17,388,600 livres

Nota Bene: As the *Kept women* of the two last Corridors are priced at a much lower rate, one does not mention *Nights* or *Fines*, which create an object of Receipt much superior to that diminution.

The MAINTENANCE of each of the girls from the six Corridors can rise, each year, because of clothing, *(in Paris)* to... 500 livres which will add up, each year, to the sum of 7,885,000 livres.

That of the chosen *Outmoded*, at 300 livres... 369,000 livres.

The cost to board the Girls, Governesses, Mistresses of Arts (per day) at 1 livres, 17,000 persons (per year)... 6,241,500 livres.

The ordinary maintenance of Buildings in all the Realm, 50,000 livres.

Sum Total... 14,545,500 livres.

N.B. this does not include a reduction for *Kept women* whom their lovers can dress, nourish, etc.

The clothing and nourishment of male and female Workers will be offset by their work. It is for this reason that I have not at all included that addition in the *Article of Receipts*. For the same reason, I have made no mention of the purchase of thread, silk, and wool necessary for the manufacture of stuffs, and the *fashion* of their habits. That ought to be found sufficiently offset by the considerable reduction that the savings on fashion will bring to the cost of clothing, and the fabrication of Stuffs.

It is worth noting that one employs only 9,585 girls out of 17,000; however, so that the Establishment will be composed almost equally of *kept women* and *prostitutes*, there will be much more revenue than I make note of; and one may consider the total *Receipts* as being a third lower than it normally comes to; while that deriving from ordinary *Maintenance* is supposedly as high as it can go in houses where the multitude of mouths will necessarily reduce the expenditure on each individual.

Consequently, that leaves, after all levied expenditures, for the Establishment, a sum much greater than... 2,743,100 livres, in excess of expenses in my hypothesis.

Which will pay for the cures for patients, wet nurses, the expenses of girls born in the house; those who can be will be married with dowries; which leaves enough to maintain the unproductive *Outmoded*.

9,585 girls will be able to give, altogether in one year, 4000 children who will live one *year* (more or less, as one will see; for of those thousands of children that die each year, many survive only a single day, others a week, or a month, &c.), *three thousand* will live *three years* (and that is a lot); and *two thousand* will attain *adolescence*; at *six livres* per month each child, in the *first year*, the *Parthénions* of the entire Realm will be responsible for 288,000 livres; the second year, one and half times that, or 450,000 livres about; the *third year*, about 576,000 livres; at the end of 8 years, about 1,200,000 livres; the rate of that burden will remain at about 1,500,000 livres, given that as the children grow older, they will cease to be a burden on the house, either by leaving it, or by their labor. One still takes here the worst case scenario; for one supposes that no father will be found who wishes to raise his children. There would remain then in that last hypothesis 1,243,100 livres, for the *Outmoded* and marriages. But I have demonstrated that the surplus of Receipts ought to be much higher.

Let's summarize: this is an almost infallible method for wiping out the *Venereal leaven*, for chasing from Europe that monster that was not made for our climate; for diminishing the scandal of Prostitution; for stopping the indecency of mores dead in its tracks; and, by supererogation, for setting up a breeding ground of subjects in the State, who will not directly depend on it; and on whom it will have an unlimited power, as paternal rights will find themselves reunited with those of the Sovereign.

I repeat: this plan would not be put into practice without some inconveniences: Prostitution, which is only tacitly tolerated, would appear authorized. That inevitable drawback, is it really real? and if it is, is it not found to be sufficiently compensated for? The one will create an effective good, and the evil will be no more than speculative, so to speak. But honestly, what is there that has no drawbacks? I wish someone could cite me an enterprise, a law, the forgiveness of wrongs even, that so sacred law that puts *Socrates* above all other men, and which a God has given us more heroic and more respectable models of; I wish someone could cite for me just one, which is not his own, and about which one cannot say sometimes[79]:

> *Quam mala sunt vicina bonis! errore sub illo*
> *pro vitio virtus crimina sæpe tulit.*[80] [81]

* * *

Madame des Tianges scolds me, my dear friend: she tells me that I should not spend so much time writing; my darling spouse seconds her: I am afraid to upset them: I will end my Letter here...

* * *

At this moment, one hears the sound of a post chaise in the courtyard: Madame Des Tianges hurries to open a casement window: "There he is, ah! there he is!" she exclaimed. And without saying anything else, she flew downstairs to be before her husband.

Monsieur Des Tianges, frightened by the Letter from his friend's uncle, had found the means to hasten his return. It is impossible to paint the joy that

---

[79]Original footnote: Crates of Thebes, a disciple of Diogenes, has given a beautiful example of moderation, that Christians have rarely imitated: A certain *Nicodrome* administered him a slap with such violence that his cheek swelled: Crates contented himself with writing at the bottom of his swollen cheek: "THIS WAS DONE BY THE HAND OF NICODROME; *Nicodromus fecit*:" a pleasant and tranquil reference to the custom of Painters. That was that poor, misshapen Crates, whom the celebrated *Hipparchia* did not blush to love, after he had sold all his possessions, the money from which he threw into the sea, crying: "*I'm free.*"

[80]Original scholium: Ovid, *de Remedio* [*Remedia Amoris*], W. 323.4

[81]*Quam... tulit*: Latin for "How very near evil is to good, by which crime often mistakes virtue for vice."

that happy arrival caused: it was all the more vivid as it succeeded the most bitter sorrow. Love, friendship, and gratitude greeted Des Tianges as he got out of the carriage: he saw his dear D'Alzan, as happy as himself; he sees him continuing to follow the path of virtue, loving his wife constantly, and meriting his happiness.

Notes

The Pornographer (or Prostitution Reformed)

Part Two

Note A. The State of Prostitution Among the Ancients

One would be much mistaken by imagining that debauchery or a predilection for pleasure were the first causes of *Prostitution*. That state, as vile as it is unfortunate and corrupt amongst us, had a less criminal origin that its effects. Not one of the false Religions admitted it into its cults:[82] it had preceded the sacrifices of human blood, which were much more atrocious. Never have men been so depraved as to believe that crime could honor Divinity: *Prostitution* was not, then, a debauchery at first, but a *consecration* from the first instant of existence of the new creature one gave life to. *Population* was the second motive for the ancient *prostitution* of girls, and even women. Such was, at least, the motive of the *Lacedaemonian* community; and, consequently, the goal of that unpublished law by Julius Caesar, which was supposed to allow women *to give themselves to as many men as they wanted*. But a devotional practice like that of *Prostitution* was bound to degenerate quickly into vice. That is what happened. The priests at first abused it to satisfy their passions. One saw the begin ning then of those despicable customs, of prostituting oneself either for the maintenance of a Temple or to amass a dowry; one saw men mutilate themselves,

---

[82]Original scholium: See *The Religions of the World* by Alexandre Ross.

thus running counter to the goal of the primitive cult: soon human blood was flowing, and one took away life instead of giving it. And that is how the two extremes came together: our Monks were set up to be poor, humble, mortified, and chaste.

Prostitution, properly speaking, which succeeds *religious prostitution*, ought not to exist except in regulated nations, where the two sexes are more or less equally free; for among those where the feebler sex is a slave, the strong makes it satisfy its pleasures, its caprices; but one cannot say that a woman, constrained by necessity, prostitutes herself. She is not, besides, for the first man who comes along; she does not receive the law except from a single man; a piece of money is not the motive that decides her: her condition consequently is less despicable. By consequence, *prostitutes* are never found in large numbers in countries known today under the names of *Turkey*, or *Persia*; I do not see anywhere that there had been prostitution in *China*; and if in some cantons of *India* the women prostituted themselves, it was a religious act, and not a vile act of commerce. I do not presume that *public women* are often seen in the deserts of *Arabia;* luxury is needed, superfluity in a nation, before one might encounter a number of those poor souls. I know that in the poorest countries, free women, or escaped or fugitive slaves, have been known to abandon themselves to every man who gave testimony to them of his desires. In the land of *Canaan*, they set themselves up as much along the public highways, as within the cities. They maintained a kind of pudor; for often they were veiled in such a way as not to be recognized; on certain occasions, they went at night to lie down at the feet of those who were resting in the country during the harvest; they remained there timidly until the moment when they were noticed. The *Bible*, which sheds some light, in passing and on the occasion of certain important events that it reports on, on the *Prostitutes* of earlier times, provides us even with information on the mores of those who were seen in Jerusalem and in the entire country of Israel, under the successor Kings of *David*. It appears that these latter were among the kind of women whose temperament led them: they sought out the most vigorous men: that did not prevent them from demanding a very considerable price (this proves that they were small in number). "She is not a Prostitute," said Ezekiel, "who does not demand payment."[83] The names that responded, in Arabic, to those of *Laïs, Thaïs, Chioné, Phryné* in Greek; to *Quartilla, Lesbia, Gallia* in Latin; were אהולה Aholah, and אהוליבה Aholibah; one must agree that these names are very expressive. As for prostitution among the young Madianite girls in the desert, one must regard it merely as a political ploy, put into practice by a people who felt too weak, in order to soften the stronger. It is in that way that unfortunate Nations of the New World have often offered the enjoyment of their women and girls to the Europeans who frightened them: thus in our own days, the sad Lapps, ashamed of their small size, engage the foreigner whom they receive to procure from him children of a less feeble and less imperfect species.

---

[83]She is not a Prostitute...: "in that thou givest a reward, and no reward is given unto thee, therefore thou art contrary [to a prostitute]." See Ezekiel, 16:34.

One must distinguish among the ancient Greeks four types of *public women*: common Prostitutes, lodged in dark houses, and whom men went to see in secret. *Girls raised into prostitution*, by the *Mastropos*[84] or *Lenon,* who had bought them, whose slaves they were, who trafficked in their charms, and who rented or sold them to whoever wanted them. *Priestesses consecrated to the cult of Venus*, who offered the sacrifice of their pudicity every day to the goddess, with the man who had chosen them, and for whom it was not permitted them to show their repugnance. There was one of those temples in Corinth. The fourth type, and without question the most famous, is the famous *Courtesans*, the *Delormes* of their century, the *Bacchae,* the *Doric,* the *Laïs,* the *Phryné,* all as well known as Alexander is in the universe. I do not say anything about the *Cytherean* girls, today *Curgo*, who prostituted themselves to foreigners along the sea shore, near the Temple of Venus, and who bore then the price of their favors and placed it on the altar to that goddess; nor those who gave themselves before marriage to the first man who came along, in order to amass their dowry (*Christopher Columbus* had not yet discovered *Haiti,* fortunately for those poor virgins!), nor the women of *Babylon,* who gave themselves, once in their life, to the man who found them to his liking: this falls under religious Prostitution; it was an accepted custom by the laws of the State. Later, they prostituted themselves to Foreigners; for that, the women remained seated in the Temple of *Nilitta,* or *Venus,* and offered themselves. They procured, by offering their favors, con-

---

[84]*Mastropos*: a pimp, proxenete, or procurer.

siderable sums, for the maintenance of the goddess' cult. Among all the ancient peoples, who gave to Divinity their most precious possession, women's sacrifice of virginity and pudicity belonged to the public and secret cult. What could have been the primitive sanctity of those sacrifices, later become abominable! A woman, in honor of the Father of Nature, before him, in his Temple, was obliged to give her life; in consequence, all the troubles of pregnancy, all the difficulties of maternity were imperative. That sacrifice, far and away greater than that of sterile *Vestals*, shows how mankind can abuse the best of things. Men, on their side, not content with participating in women's homage, pushed extravagance to the point of banging their heads against the primitive intention, by depriving themselves of their virility, an abusive sacrifice from the get-go; deplorable effect of false ideas that one began to have of Divinity.

Among the Romans, who had taken their Religion from the Greeks, it was rather ordinary to see them change the practices. *Religious prostitution* no longer had a place; the cult of *Phallus* or *Priapus* became ridiculous. Among the Republicans, then, one saw *Prostitutes* only of the first two types that we have distinguished in Greece. With them, legitimate *Concubinage* had for a long time replaced *Prostitution*. At home, a man found all that could satisfy the variety of his desires. However, their Lupanaria were more important locations than our *bad places*. In Petronius, one finds ample description of them. It appears that one abandoned oneself to all kinds of debauchery there, and that the *Meretrices* were not as ugly as the greater part of *Prostitutes* today, automatons moved by money, who neither move nor feel as soon as it is out of sight. There was at all times in Rome a quarter for *public women*. They did not mix with Citizens. In those miserable times, when *Caligula*, *Nero*, *Commodus* and their like placed impudence on the throne; when Roman Ladies no longer knew neither modesty nor restraint; the *Prostitutes retained a kind of decency*; the following Epigram by *Martial* proves it:

> *Incustoditis & apetis, Lesbia, semper*
>   *Liminibus peccas, nec tua furta tegis*
> *Et plus specator quam te delectat adulter,*
>   *Nec sunt grata tibi guadia si qua latent:*
> *At Meretrix Abigit Testem Veloque Serâque,*
>   *Raraque Summœni[85] rima patet:*
> *A Chione saltem vel Laïde disce pudorem,*
>   *Abscondunt spurcas & monumenta Lupas.*
> *Numquid dura tibi nimiùm censura videtur?*
>   *Deprendi veto te, Lesbia...*

Nothing equaled the cleanliness of Greek and Roman *Courtesans*; they gave to the maintenance of their bodies an attention worthy of the praise men made of their beauty; they employed all means imaginable to enhance the whiteness of their skin, to conserve the splendor and freshness of their charms; those means were the unctuous ointments they used to cover their faces, their hands, their neck, their bosom, &c. at night; baths, which became then an absolute

---

[85]Original scholium: *Summœni*: as if to say *a place situated under the city walls*: it was, in ancient Rome, a quarter near the ramparts, set aside for public women.

necessity; depilatories, &c. One sees in the statues that we have still from Antiquity that they did not keep even that veil by which a Natural modesty hid their secret charms: perhaps it was because of the heat of the climate, for the cleanliness so essential to their sex, or, if one wishes, for the commodity of pleasure, and the voluptuousness of looks.

Those *girls* did not *become automatons* like those of our days: one does not see in Petronius, in Martial, nor in the other Authors who mention the *Prostitutes* of their times, that they had pushed stultification to the point of making themselves *insensitive.* Far from it: those Authors represent them to us as women for whom the habit of pleasure had made a necessity of sexual pleasure. We have fallen quite low compared to the Ancients in that regard. One will agree, without further elaboration, that the excesses that deprive women of *sensitivity,* by too frequent a reiteration, ought to give to the *Haitian* malady that degree of malignity that it is certain not to possess on the soil where it was born.

Present State of Prostitution

The mores of modern Nations, that the Religions they profess have made much more serious and decent than those of the Ancients, are also more contrary to *Prostitution*. Far be it from them for prostitution to be an act of their cult, – nothing is more contrary to its spirit.

It is, for men living in society, a brake more powerful than the laws, it is *opinion*; there is no state that could not respect it, there is no excess one might not be capable of, when its yoke is removed from us. Today's Religions have inspired only horror for *public women*; they have branded them, ranked them below brutes; the universe has believed to recognize in that judgment the voice of Divinity and Reason; it has applauded. Poor mortals! you are not ignorant of this, the infamy of a condition is not what makes it less numerous; and the ordinary effect of debasement that you have attached to it, what is that? Examine experience; it will show you man always placing himself below the depravation of the state that he descends to: before the contempt identified with its type of lifestyle, he would not have been half so vicious; you have found the means of turning him into a wicked scoundrel. A Cytherean girl, a Syrian, a Priestess of Venus, a Laplander lives honestly after having prostituted herself; a French woman, an English *girl of the world*, are beyond redemption, monsters that the earth ought to swallow up. The reason for this difference? It is that the first didn't believe they had debased themselves, and that the second, resolute to enter into a condition where they are sure to have nothing more to expect from their sex than a disdainful abandonment, and from all their society but a rigorous contempt, so as to render them insensitive to it, have degraded their existence through all the vices that bastardize the soul. There is nothing easier than to brand, and nothing more fatal in its effects, not only for the debased individuals, but for all mankind. If that there is a certain truth with regards to *Prostitutes*, what would I say about useful professions, such as the *Theater* for example? But one must treat of that elsewhere.

Such is *Prostitution* among modern Nations. It is a vile state, grown contrary to increasing the population, that at the beginning it had to favor; destructive of good behavior; dangerous for health, for life even, whose sources it attacks; practiced by famished *she-wolves* for whom nothing is sacred, and who pay us back, with usury, all the evil that the Laws make for them; and those are also the inconveniences that the Pornographer seeks to diminish.

Vilified, branded, chased, punished, often inhumanely, *Prostitutes* are more numerous now than ever before; it is a sad truth, impermissible to doubt of. But what were the causes of the renaissance of *modern Prostitution*, which the subservience of almost all Nations by the Barbarians of the North had made disappear rather broadly? The extreme *inequality* that had lulled it, reproduced it: the Nobles, by their despicable *Culetage,*[86] *Jambage,*[87] and *Prelibation,*[88] took from their Vassals the first flower of the integrity of mores. Sullied by her Master, a young woman often abandoned herself to others. The progress of vice is rapid. *Prostitution* reappeared.

---

[86]*Culetage*: or *couletage*, a synonym of *courtage* possibly; a fixed tax on the sale or purchase of merchandise.

[87]*Jambage*: the right of a seigneur to the leg of each slaughtered cow.

[88]*Prelibation*: a custom by which a seigneur could sleep with the bride of a vassal on the first wedding night.

Let's cast a glance at all known nations: there are none that *Prostitution* has not sullied, and where the *Haitian* malady has not followed.

Public women are rarer in Asiatic Principalities than in Christian nations; for reasons that I have already given; one finds them however in large cities of the Orient, principally in those that a seaport makes more commercial and more frequented by Foreigners: these are unfortunate souls, those Greek girls debased by Mussulmen. Jews, European navigators, native Christians of that country are the only ones who visit them; that is why Venereal diseases are very rare in the States of the Grand-Seignior[89] and other Potentates of Asia. Muslim women do not prostitute themselves: but do their mores gain thereby? Far from it: Turks of a limited fortune being unable to visit a Christian prostitute, without risk to their life and that of the public women, have recourse to even more shameful remedies.

I have almost nothing to say about America. *Prostitution* is still practiced there, among the subdued natives, as part of their cult: the Colonies have the mores of the Nations they depend on; the Slaves do the will of their Master: the women of free Savages follow the instincts of nature. The malady of the *Antilles* is endemic in certain cantons in that part of the world; but the cure is relatively facile. Among the *Peruvians*, the *Mexicans*, and the *inhabitants of the civilized Isles, religious* Prostitution had degenerated

---

[89]Grand-Seignior: the sultan of Turkey.

into debauchery at the time of discovery of their countries: the two sexes were even accused of pederasty before the Spanish Council, and that was one of the apparent motives for the barbarous order that was given to exterminate them: I doubt, despite those indications, that Americans practiced the profession of *Prostitution*: it is almost certain that they did not abandon themselves to every man except on certain occasions, and that they resumed the ordinary way of life afterwards. That conduct is still today something that women of the California peninsula practice, at the festival of *Skins* and at that of the *Pitahaya* harvest.

It is then in Europe that one must strive to see the *Prostitution of women*, in all the turpitude and infamy that must accompany a condition that Religion and the Laws equally reprove; followed by the disorders and dangers that it brings with it.

London would be the city in Europe that could do best without public *Prostitutes* and for this reason: the mores of a portion of the women are nothing less than severe; *Taverns*, where the two sexes can equally assemble without scandal, offer to those who want to satisfy too active a penchant for pleasure, a commodity that one does not find so easily anywhere else; despite that relaxation of mores, the number of Prostitutes there is not any smaller; their impudence, which goes to extremes, strikes one all the more, as the honest women of the three Realms are of a modesty and restraint that inspires respect, tenderness, and never audacity. The division into classes, that will be found hereinafter in the article on *Paris*, can equally serve for the Capital of Great Britain.

In *Germany, public women* are tolerated in large cities, and chased from smaller ones as soon as they are found out. One could say that that country, and *Switzerland*, are, in Europe, those that have preserved innocence the most: no other disorder replaces *Prostitution* there. Let's not give them too much credit though: if they had large cities, if one saw immense fortunes and too much inequality among those peoples, corruption would be communicated immediately: there are cantons in France, where the mores are pure; and cities in Germany, like Berlin, that go further than Paris and London in terms of disorder. The temperature of a climate is but a weak barrier, in opposition to the corruption of some men, whom the affluence of all pleasures holds in infatuation, and who cannot reawaken their dulled senses except by paying their weight in gold for despicable indulgences. Venereal illnesses and their cure were almost unknown in Germany before the last two wars: the Swiss would still be a disinterested spectator of the general plague, if some of its children, who put themselves into the pay of their powerful neighbors, hadn't brought the poison back to their mother's breast. But one says that in the last several years, libertinage is spreading, and that examples of the most shameful disorders become less rare. (Depravation follows the progress of enlightenment. A very natural thing, that men cannot become enlightened without being corrupted: their organs become more delicate, the perfected soul sees farther, has more varied desires; in that new condition, new pleasures are needed; Natural ones are too simple: one complicates them in order to give them some spice; but all that one adds to Nature leads to disorder, and becomes criminal. It is neither Religion nor Laws that can change anything in that march of the mores; like a river fattened by melting snows, it breaks open the powerless dikes that only serve to add more fury to their overflowing. Barbarity, and excess of wit in a Nation, are equally dangerous reefs for its mores. When, as in Berlin, England, Italy, France, one is in the second case, one must suffer a little disorder. It is an unfortunate necessity, which can be compared to the retreat that an able General is forced sometimes to make: never can it dishonor a Government. A rule as perfect as it is impossible, given the present mores, would be that young people marry as soon as they are adults. I see only the villages where that could be practiced without too much inconvenience. It is not easy for everyone to imagine all manner of debauchery that the corruption of great cities suggests to men deprived of all natural means to satisfy their needs of temperament: it is what makes me unafraid to advance that a *Parthénion* would be useful in every city that houses Troops; the injunction against marrying, that military discipline makes necessary, would cease to be hard for soldiers, and would no longer expose them to the corrupting influence of tramps, one or two sufficing to empoison an entire regiment. One could choose for cities of war, those very large and very well-made German *prostitutes*; by that means our most handsome men would not live in vain for posterity.) Coming back to the matter of small German towns: they are in the same situation as our second-order provincial cities, where one sees only *Prostitutes in passing,* and the most often Miserable wretches, like those of the *Twelfth Class* in the Capital.

Courtesans have a quarter in Christian *Rome*, as formerly they had in Sommenie; there are some among them who show great feelings combined with a rare beauty; these latter choose their world, give themselves over to honest men only, and keep scruples about receiving several men, when a single one suffices for them to procure life's necessities. In which they differ greatly from the *kept girls* of Paris and London, who advertise themselves as being attached to a single man, and who go with whomever pleases them or pays for them. There is yet another variety in *Naples*, in *Florence*, and in the principle cities of *Italy*: very young women place themselves under the guidance of an Older Woman, known by *Monsignori* and old voluptuous Seigneurs; that woman introduces them each evening to a rich Old Man, who sends them away after he has satisfied his rather strange fantasies with them. If the debauched old man himself pays, the young woman is quit of those humiliating indulgences; but if his main Domestic is charged with paying her, he demands, while acquitting his commission, the same as his master, and sometimes more. As soon as the charms of those unfortunate girls have lost their initial freshness, they no longer have any resource but to give themselves over to the public.

Spanish prostitutes are, of all Europeans, those who practice their vile profession the most seriously. The natural ferocity of their Nation exposes them daily to a thousand brutal fantasies, which degrade them more than anywhere else. It would be dangerous to cite some examples. But the unfortunate inhabitant of Mexico and the mountains of *San Luis Postosí* would be avenged, if he saw the sisters and daughters of his tyrants submitted to their caprices... There is perhaps no other country in the world where the human species is more corrupt. The girls, shut up in their paternal house, where they have seen no men other than their brothers, leave it sullied to pass into the arms of their husbands... (One notes however that the natural gentleness of the house of *Bourbon* begins to temper that atrocity of mores imprinted on the Nation by the Pèdres, the Philippes II, the Dukes of Albe, &c.)

I will give details, under the article on *French prostitutes*, which I have merely abridged to give space for other Nations.

One can divide them into *twelve Classes*:

1. *Girls Kept by a single man, who do not hesitate to give him Associates.* This *first* Class is at a rate that one cannot determine: it procures pleasures that are not always certain.

2. *Public Girls by Status: such are the Chorus Girls, Dancers in Operas, &c.* This class is the most dangerous. (I do not mentioned famous Actresses, and that out of respect for the virtue of several among them.) They ruin Marquis, Dukes, Lords; they even drain Financiers.

3. *The Demi-Kept Girls: these are the young*

women taken at a public Madame's, that a man found pretty enough to want to take care of. This class is less to be feared, but it is vile, and unworthy of a delicate man. The demi-kept girls require only a tidy bourgeois maintenance. (Our amusing books are filled with the tricks that have been played and are played without cease on their dupes by these first three classes. Everything has been said about Girls of the Theater, and those young innocents to whom one gives a small or large house. But I have to add that Greek satyr scenes, however bloody they might appear on stage, have never come close to the truth: I have witnessed over and beyond what I have read. But I will spare *Kept Women* the details, in favor of their demi-integrity. Nevertheless, one will allow me to say of these girls of the third class that it is not so flattering to take charge of a girl whom a thousand others have defiled; who, like Turkish or Persian slaves, is faithful only while waiting for the occasion not to be. How can one dare to go outside with her, to show one's face at Spectacles, at Promenades, where one is at every moment singled out? Is it not natural to have a bad opinion of a man who braves all that? It remains to be seen in each article, on the manner in which that vile commerce is exercised, which serves to disabuse men who are rather happy for not knowing it by experience. One will see that one cannot enjoy true pleasures with the poor souls I speak of. There is no means surer to inspire in the two sexes a just horror of debauchery. Vice, in and of itself, is so ugly that it always frightens, from the moment one presents it without the ornaments that a corrupt imagination knows how to attribute to it.)

4. *Girls of Average-Virtue, who prostitute themselves only in* the interim, *in their regular profession's off seasons, with the sole view of meeting pressing needs.* The girls here in question span all the inferior classes; they have no specific rank. (They could be excusable if that were possible while embracing such a condition.) (Libertines make a ragout with girls of this class, when they succeed in discovering one. In what does that vaunted pleasure consist for them? To triumph over a girl who languishes in necessity; who devours her tears while caressing you, and behold the most honest among them, or even, a shameless hussy, who is reduced to the height of humiliation in order to earn her daily bread, to tell the truth, but without repugnance for the crime, as without taste for the pleasure; moreover, often coarse, unsavory? Oh! sad, detestable sensual pleasure!)

5. *Courtesans, who make a number of acquaintances, who receive them and who go to visit them.* Libertines of a limited fortune make different arrangements amongst themselves, which this class of girl lends itself to. I could cite some examples that strike fear in the heart of the virtuous Citizen. It is said that young

Female Laborers, still living at home, have had two, three, and even as many as six *Friends* at a modest price per week. (This class of girl offers to libertinage something more spicy, and less fastidious; always proper, elegant even; ordinarily what one might call *sensible* in debauchery terms, they can touch the heart, but never the soul, never; the power of their attractions does not go that deep. Eh! what is love, when reduced to love of the senses?... O unfortunate girls, be honest, let your heart be softened for an inestimable object, and I will be the judge of your case. You enjoy it, do you say? Insane, and what exactly?... You tremble! There is no more time, the poison ingested yesterday circulates today in your veins!... and you deserve it.)

6. *High-Society Women, to whom Old Women bring Johns, and who, when they go out, do not advertise their status.* One is particularly fond, in this class, of moderately debauched Old Men.

7. *Madame's Girls, who are set aside for Old Men, or others, who pay dearly. They are sometimes escorted into the country to the houses of wealthy Libertines.*

8. *The Demure and Fashionable Ones. This class, as well as that of the Madames, have more than one use. Both are a dangerous stumbling block for people needing reserve.* The girls in this category, ordinarily of a certain age, are a bit more reasonable than the

others; they show more restraint in their conduct, hold themselves well, have a vile man whom they call a *Friend*, which word those despicable mouths deem it proper to profane, as they have acted for a long time as a *Lover*.

9. *The Hussies.*[90] *These girls live like those of the seventh class, living with Madames; but they take the first man who comes along, and they fend for themselves. They run from one bad place to another.* These ill-fated wretches lead a very sordid and extremely sad life, without much profit for themselves, their *Madames* paying for their pensions, clothes, and the linen they rent to them, rather expensively, such that they have nothing left over, while exposing their health at every instant for those vile beings; often they extort something by dint of solicitations; the surplus from it is all theirs.

10. *The Whores.*[91] *They are rather poorly lodged in furnished rooms, and subject to no small number of inconveniences by the police. They sometimes live with the Madames of their class. The lot of them live in a state of great insecurity.* Nothing proves more clearly to what point passion leads us astray than the courage that some well-bred men have to follow a miserable wretch from the dregs of society into a dirty hovel where they dare to sit

---

[90]Hussies: *Boucaneuses* in French.

[91]Whores: *Rachrocheuses* in French.

down. In order to satisfy their brute nature, they are presented with an unclean and even unhealthier object: everything one sees there disgusts; and if it is possible that a creature of this class had any charms, her behavior, her manners quickly destroy any illusion. O mortals! do you want to see humanity at the lowest rung of its degradation, follow one of those miserable wretches into her dirty den; a thinking man will have nothing there to fear from his passions; he will experience a feeling of sorrow and pity mixed with indignation.

11. *The Gouines[92]: they are dressed in a "casaquin" or small dress, and are ordinarily rather disgusting.* The girls of this class go a little bit beyond those of the tenth: one is surprised sometimes that such monsters can get along at the expense of men.

12. *The Street-Walkers: These are the miserable wretches that are found along buildings and in unfrequented streets; who have for a lodging a hovel in the faubourgs, where they do not bring anybody ordinarily. They are very dangerous for manual laborers whom they rope in, and whom they infect with their Venereal poison.* These miserable wretches need a more vile name: ugly, disgusting, sordid, they attract however the attention of a pack of poor Artisans, Locksmiths, Knife Sharpeners, Blacksmiths, Masons, Manual Laborers, Wa-

---

[92]Original scholium: this word comes from the English word "Queen" (quoine), which is given to them in derision.

ter Bearers, &c. who are not married. (One must include in the same tableau these last seven classes of workers. Excitable by temperament, moved by the constant view of women who please him; a man feels disquieting, pressing, often impetuous desires stirring in him: in spite of himself, despite reason, nature seeks to be satisfied; at that moment, he goes to see a Prostitute; he finds the same charms that attracted him: his imagination paints the pleasures of nature to him; he feels transported; he is flattered to think that those who excite him share in his excitement: he accosts them; his reception by these despicable women is almost always sweet; he follows them; he is cajoled by them until the moment he pays; but if he takes too long, he is pressured; from the moment the Prostitute has received her wages, her only concern is one thing, that of promptly getting rid of the man. If sometimes, a rather pretty mouth appears to ask for a kiss, a revolting breath soon repels him. Her heart, always made of ice, her impatience when she sees herself too tormented, would chase Venus away from *Paphos* or *Cythera*. But, grant her one last favor, and it is then that the danger becomes greatest, and when nature, gravely offended even in her very sanctuary, punishes criminal voluptuousness... Such are French Prostitutes then, and here you have the seductive bait they present! Even if one were quit for having paid so dear, without experiencing the kind of satisfaction one was promised! but almost always a cold sensual pleasure has frightening consequences: one is punished for the pleasure one did not enjoy; the regrets must be more bitter still.

M. de Voltaire proposes, in jest, a method for getting rid of the virus, by employing against it the 1,200,000 standing troops that Europe keeps during peace time. One could at least make use of them to conduct a search as exact as it is strict of all Prostitutes, to oblige them to be housed in the Parthénions. Two advantages would result from that reform: the virus would disappear imperceptibly: prostitution would day after day become rarer; and who knows? it could die out altogether at length.

When Venereal Disease began to manifest itself in Europe, one considered it a kind of plague; a Judgment dated March 6, 1496,[93] forbade people suffering from the Pox, under pain of capital punishment, any interaction with healthy persons. They were given alms, and they were sequestered like Lepers.

---

[93]March 6, 1496: the attentive reader will notice this date as only 3.5 years after the date on which Christopher Columbus discovered the Americas.

Note B

Women among the ancient Greeks and Romans did not live as Women among the French or English do; one is familiar with the severity of the laws that *Romulus* imposed on them. It was reserved doubtless to the two most illustrious and enlightened Nations that have ever existed, to render unto the prettier half of the human race rights too long usurped from them. These Nations have surpassed the very famous piety of Romans with respect to their mothers and their wives: to treat them as equals is much greater than responding to their prayers, or protecting them. That reasonable behavior brings the two sexes together, strengthens the bonds that unite them, and seems to have banished the shameful vices that infected the Greeks and Romans, vices that their own Authors sought to make them blush for. See Martial, Epigrams 51 Book II; 71, 73 and 75 Book II; 50 book IV; 45 Book VIII; 7 book IX; 25 book XI. Petronius, Juvenal, Suetonius, &c.

Honest women can, by themselves, prevent a large number of disorders, inevitable without them; everything speaks in their favor; they have their charms, more provoking than beauty; when they stop being so air-headed and demanding; when they are sincere, tender, less changeable, more *sensitive;* they will submit everything to the invincible charm of those attractions destined by Nature to captivate us; and we will owe them, with a real felicity, the integrity of our mores.

Note C

From among the many examples that a young Physician has furnished to me, I am going to choose one, while suppressing personally identifying details.

…A young man, who was established in this city for several years, came to take me on a walk with him. We were traversing S*** bridge... when a very pretty woman passed by us, accompanied by a well-dressed man, and who appeared to be still in the flower of youth. The beauty of that Lady struck us. In the evening, we found ourselves in front of a Convent of Venus... My friend, who at that time still was not a model of wisdom, held a conversation with the Abbess. After a moment, he rejoined me, and explained to me what I had mistaken for an ordinary acquaintance: he told me that she was arranging for him one of those adventures that are not known anywhere else but in the Capitals, and that he was going to visit her that same evening. I did what I could to dissuade him, and to inspire in him a just horror of those despicable places. But seeing him obstinate in his resolution, I left him rather early.

In the middle of the night, I was told that someone was knocking very strongly at the door. I ordered that it be opened, and I arranged to have myself dressed, when my imprudent friend presented himself to my view, but entirely beside himself; he was pale, haggard, downcast; he could barely hold himself up: his condition frightened me. I gave him some cordials and had him put to bed. On reawakening, he recounted to me his adventure; and it was with the utmost surprise that I learnt from his mouth that he had spent the night in a place that he named for me, with that same woman whom we were admiring the day before.

The Plan that I am putting together will destroy the unhappy facility with which they may satisfy themselves, the women who abandon themselves to such shameful disorders.

Note D

The young man mentioned in the previous Note recounted to his friend that, one day, at around five o'clock in the evening, *** followed, on a whim, an Old Woman into a place of debauchery... He quickly noticed that the young woman who was presented to him was not of the convent. He made different attempts to get to know her... As chance would have it, he saw her leave one day from her parents' house at around nine o'clock in the morning, a prayer book under her arm; he flies after her in pursuit; she enters a Church rapidly, files out into a small side street, and slips into... the Old Woman's place.

The young man saw her several times in the same way... But he does not enjoy his so-called good fortune for as long as he would have liked. One day as he was passing, according to his habit, into the street of that chaste person, he noticed many carriages in front of her door. At ten o'clock, he saw her exit the house elegantly dressed, beautiful as an angel, adorned as the symbol of purity: she was going to swear an eternal oath to a young lover, who appeared drunk on his good fortune...[94]

---

[94] *Dicis formosam, dicis te, Bassa, puellam;/Istud qua non est dicere Bassa solet.* [Latin for "You say Bassa, that you are a beautiful girl;/Something that is not a normal thing to say, Bassa."] – Martial L. V. Epigram 46. This lie is no longer fashionable; our girls never talk about themselves.

Note E

A man was introduced into a place of debauchery by one of those women who greet passersby. On his arrival, there was a big commotion in the house; of the sort that he found it impossible to exit, and it was not prudent for him to show himself. That particular man took the advice of the girl who had led him there; he retired into a small room, whose door with a window gave onto another room where several libertines were gathered around two very young, very fetching women, whom they had made undress... They were tied up... A cruel precaution stifled their cries... (Here, I leave out certain revolting circumstances...) They pushed their barbarousness too far, so that fearing the Abbess and the girl who had just entered the room would go call out for help, they bound both the latter to the foot of the bed. The unfortunate man who had come to that accursed house to find pleasure, shuddered in horror. He witnessed a thousand monstrous and degrading things... Finally that cruel spectacle ended. But before exiting, those despicable persons had the inhumanity of pricking lightly with their swords the two poor souls who were at their mercy. They could not cry out loud, but instead a heavy groaning was heard; which had something terrifying about it; one saw the tears flowing profusely down their cheeks, and mixing with their drops of blood...

Note F

One could make some very fine arguments for the hability of *constantly loving* either one object or another, particularly of the human species. Whoever envis-
ages *love* as a liniment that is always ready, not only,
like friendship, to soften our troubles, but to suspend
our feelings of them, to efface any impression of
them, to destroy them entirely; *love*, I say, considered
from that angle, is clearly the most precious gift Divinity could give, and the antidote of a sad and far-
sighted reason. Man has the misfortune of knowing
that he will die: he has even the pride of thinking that
of all living creatures he is the only one who knows it
(and so much the better for the poor animals, who do
not have the same means we do to be stunned by it).
He has then two additional needs than they do: that of
living in society, so that the sight of others like himself might almost always distract him, that their example might encourage and console him; and that of a
feeling that infuses a kind of intoxication in his heart
when forced to enter it. Love's natural intoxication, as
much as, and more so than that of wine, than that of
glory, than the seething transports of fury, makes him
despise death: feeling the most violent or the most unreasonable passions is useful to us and necessary
against our feeble reason. Oh! what preservatives we
would need if, for example, its lights allowed us to
see into the future! Our bodies would need a stronger
constitution; vegetables and other aliments destined to
maintain our life would need to contain stronger
juices; the entire system of nature would be changed;

that is to say our globe would no longer be as it is, what it is, or where it is, and we would need to be greater than men; otherwise the shock of necessary passions for equilibrium would destroy our organs. *Our lights come up so short!* so the most enlightened of men tell us; while a coarse peasant believes his own to be as expansive as they can possibly be: as much to say that the latter man is in a natural place for man – below nature; and that the former has risen above it; the peasant is a child at the bottom of a valley, who thinks he sees all the universe, and that the hills touch the clouds; the scholar[95] is a made man, at the summit of the Alps, who discovers an immense horizon, and who is irritated that the weakness of his organs let him merely perceive what he would want to distinguish. The happier of the two? Reason would say the peasant. A question that presents itself is to know whether the manner of living, in civilized nations, has not extended the hability to love; whether the laws of modesty, the graces that adornment add to a woman's beauty, the *succulence* of aliments, – have not made that faculty continuous? That's my opinion at any rate.

"A celebrated Philosopher of our days examines in his *Natural History* why love makes all creatures happy, but man unhappy. He responds that *there is in that passion merely a physical good; and the mental good, that is to say the* feeling, *that accompanies it, is worthless.* That Philosopher did not claim that the mental good does not add to physical pleasure, experience would prove otherwise; nor that the

---

[95]scholar: in 2021, we would say "scientist."

mental good of love is merely an illusion, which is true, but does not destroy the vivacity of pleasure (eh, how few pleasures have a real object!); clearly, what he wanted to say was that the mental good is what causes all the harm of love; and in this, we could not agree with him more. Let us conclude only that if lights superior to reason did not allow us a better condition, we would have a strong argument for complaining about Nature, which, while presenting to us on the one hand the most seductive of pleasures, seems to push us away on the other, by the dangers, of every sort, with which it is surrounded, and which have, so to speak, placed us on the edge of a precipice, between grief and privation."

Let us justify Nature and Love; neither the first nor the second are to be blamed; it is still *inequality* that has caused all the trouble: perfectly equal among themselves, animals love without preference; youth and the beauty of form, in females, adds nothing to the eagerness of males. It is certain, by the knowledge that we have of the mores of certain peoples of America, that it must have been the same with early man: every woman was good to them; this latter, by a feeling particular to her sex, always defended herself a little, then submitted finally to her victor. All was limited then to the appetite of the senses, and man, far from gaining thereby, lost two-thirds of his happiness. But a sweeter feeling, hidden in his soul, struggled to develop: beauty must have given birth to it; among those wretched creatures who find their subsistence with difficulty, such as, for example, *Californians*, that advantage does not exist; can Venus and the Graces caress a gaunt face that has ardent, disquieted eyes; a complexion, a neck covered with dust, burnt in the sun, and become scaly almost by the intemperance of the seasons? Beauty must have begun to distinguish women only when the human species had need of it. That was when the taste for preference was born, which alone, since then, has borne the name of love. But the choice was for a long time the privilege of the male; the timid sex, content to see in him, to whom she was given, her defender and her support, had no other penchant than her duty. Calm spectator to the battle between two fierce rivals, and sure to have a hero for a spouse, *Deianira* would have loved *Alcides*, the victor of *Achelous*. The two primary sources of inequality between men were Religion and Heroism: the deference that one had for the first Priests, as interpreters of the Gods, soon became submission: Heroes, particularly bold, unjust, and wicked, brought about the degradation of humankind: they extorted by fear the same homages that persuasion caused to be given to Ministers of Divinity: those who wanted to defend themselves against it were pushed down even lower, they were made into Slaves. Here we find ourselves arrived at the lowest rung of inequality: affluence reigns, the disproportion of fortunes is immense, beauty shines from the freshness of repose, from the sparkle of satisfaction and that of adornment: the Slave, to whom, of all the advantages of his being, nothing remains but a sensitive heart, straightening his curved back in order to wipe the sweat from his disgusting brow, he sees the daughter of his tyrant; the flowers of youth embellish her face; while he is admiring her, she casts a glance at him, an expressive mark of compassion that inspires him; the wretch lowers his gaze, and goes back to his work again: but his soul is wounded; he is consumed with unprofitable desires; the tyrant's daughter has caused him more harm than the tyrant himself, and his unhappiness is complete. One can compare the consequences of inequality, more or less, in the other ranks of fortune. But the evil becomes all of a sudden extreme when women believe themselves permitted to choose their master, on whom their modesty, from the most distant past, did not allow them to lift their eyes. Man was miserable by a feeling similar to what made him desire riches, honors, all those goods whose possession is envied, and the acquisition of which was difficult. Was that the vice of Love and the fault of Nature? No: that so-called admirable subordination of rank and fortune, so vaunted by vile adulators, is the source of all the moral evil that one sees in society! Before I finish up this note, I return to the animals: are we really certain they have no advance idea of death? I do not believe it is easy to fix the extent of it, but I think that the effort put into conserving one's life, and the idea of destruction, are inseparable. If animals recognize danger, if they flee from it, if they avoid it with skill, then they anticipate death, at minimum instantaneously and in a confused way: otherwise, whence come those bellowings of the bull, when his nostrils catch wind of an animal of his same species devoured by carnivorous beasts? What would cause excessive fright in a pig when some venomous reptile approaches, or when it hears thunderclaps? Hunters know the ruses that the fear of death instills in their prey; and I have observed that the fright of sheep, in the presence of a wolf, was so great that

their pupils glazed over and that they turned around
without seeing, for several minutes. Animals are not
as stupid as one thinks, and are more miserable because of it.

Note G

"I was summoned," a young Physician said to me some time ago, "to ***'s place, for a rather pretty girl, of my acquaintance. I was told she was dangerously ill: I presumed that her indisposition was the *usual consequence* of her miserable profession... I found her in a frightening condition... A man, whom she had just enjoyed the pleasures of love with, had tried to force her to... She absolutely refused... that maniac pinched her nipple with such force that she fainted. He left her in that state, and exited the house.

"I had her bandaged in front of me; the nipple was almost detached; the Surgeon despaired of her recovery, but I augured better of her wound, and that girl is effectively recovered. What is particularly fortunate for her is that that accident so greatly frightened her that she consented to my putting her into an apprenticeship; a proposition that she had always avoided to accept, under various pretexts."

See Martial, Epigram 79, Book II.

Note H

"A very nice and very sweet young person, whose parents I knew quite well," said again the young Physician who furnished me with the tales I have reported, "was constrained by them to marry a man who had been very debauched. He was rich, and the Demoiselle had no property. It was thus a sad example of marriages in which monetary interest alone had decided the matter. Her husband, not content with plunging himself into drunkenness, took up his old habits again. One day she had me summoned: I believed she was upset: I flew to her. Several times, during our conversation, I saw her on the verge of letting the tears fall, which tears she did her best to hold back. Moreover, she complained only of vapors, disquietudes, an involuntary sadness. I did everything I could to calm her; soon I realized that I was only making things worse. As other patients were waiting for me, I prepared to leave, when she begged me, by a thousand entreaties, to remain until her husband returned. I was as surprised by that request as I had been of her grief. We spent the rest of the day together, without her letting escape anything that could have informed me. Finally we heard her husband come home, and we knew that he was not alone. 'Ah! the miserable wretch,' said the young Lady to me then, 'he did what he threatened he would do... Monsieur,' she added, 'I know your discretion, and the integrity of your feelings. I beg you not to leave here.' At the same time, she showed me a small closet, and asked me to shut myself in it, when the hour to retire had come; she added hastily that my assistance would be necessary to her during the night. I promised to accord her that satisfaction, not knowing where any of this was going to lead. The husband appeared; a pretty person whom the most decided impudence prevented from being too pleasant, accompanied him. He appeared surprised to see me; however he made me great demonstrations of amity, and we sat down to table together. My presence avoided, during supper, a thousand mortifications that he had promised to inflict on his wife. He drank profusely, and often complained of something I could not get to the bottom of exactly. When I noticed that it was getting late, I took my leave of them. The young Lady followed me. We opened the door; but instead of exiting, I went into the closet, as we had agreed.

"No sooner was I in there than I heard, with as much surprise as indignation, him ordering his wife to offer the basest of services to that vile creature who had come to defy her; he told her that he wanted her to witness the pleasures he was going to enjoy with that contemptible rival. That poor woman obeyed, and said nothing; but when her unworthy husband was in bed, she ran to the closet where I was hiding: she spent the night there, in spite of his threats and the efforts he made to break the door down. I needed all my strength and all my skill to prevent him from succeeding. He grew discouraged, and returned to the arms of the woman he had brought with him. After that abominable man had exhausted all his brutality, he fell asleep. It was then that I asked the young Lady if such scenes occurred often, and why didn't she tell her parents? Here's what she told me:

"'You see, Monsieur, that I am the most miserable of women: but you do not yet know the half of it: my parents, who ought to console me, to protect me, my unnatural parents, anticipated by my husband, repulse me, accuse me of deceit; they refuse to assure themselves with their own eyes of the truth that I tell them: they repeat *to my husband the complaints that I made to them of his conduct, and they have caused him to mistreat me. But that is not even the worst of my problems: accustomed to seeing only those despicable creatures who sell their modesty, my husband demands from me... I was forced to escape the night before last, in order to hide from his importunateness, and I locked myself in this closet. He exited in the morning, telling me in a mocking tone of voice that he saw clearly I was in need of some lessons, which he would give to me and which would banish my stupid scruples, and that that very evening another woman, more complaisant than me to all his fantasies, would take my place; that I should consider treating her like my mistress... without you, Monsieur,' she added, 'I would have had no other recourse than to try and escape again, to wander aimlessly during the night; to avoid remaining exposed to all that a heart as corrupted as that of that tyrant would have made me endure, and the insolence of that vile creature you saw with him.'*

"I was moved by the fate of a woman as virtuous as she was kind. I led her back to her parents in the morning, while her husband was still sleeping; I painted for them a picture, in the most vivid colors, of the atrocious fate of their daughter. Nature expressed itself in their hearts; I had persuaded them; they were

moved to tears by the poor soul who had always
loved them tenderly. They agreed that she should
leave her husband without making a scene, and several days later, a Lady of condition, very respectable,
who had retired to a Convent, made herself a companion who becomes more dear to her with each passing
day."

A Roman said to his wife

Uxor, vade foras, aut moribus utere nostris:
   non sum ego nec Curius nec Numa nec
                    [Tatius.
Me jucunda juvant tractae per pocula noctes:
   tu properas pota surgere tristis aqua.
Tu tenebris gaudes: me ludere teste lucerna
   et juvat admissa rumpere luce latus.
Fascia te tunicaeque obscuraque pallia celant:
   at mihi nulla satis nuda puella jacet.
basia me capiunt blandas imitata columbas:
   tu mihi das aviae qualia mane soles.
Nec motu dignaris opus nec voce juvare...
      ... dabat hoc Cornelia Graccho,
Julia Pompeio, Porcia, Brute, tibi;...
Si te delectat gravitas, Lucretia toto
   sis licet usque die: Laida nocte volo.

— Martial L. XI Epigrams 104.

That double tableau of the innocent, frugal,

chaste life of ancient Romans, and the unconstrained conduct of the men of Nero's century, offers an admirable contrast: but at the same time, it is, I believe, reflective of what corruption of the human heart can produce of the most licentious kind. One sees in that Epigram an abuse of the greatest names combined with a blasphemy of the Gods. No, I repeat, we have not yet devolved (at least not openly) to that degree of perversity. It really needed women, although very beautiful in those distant centuries, to remain ignorant in the arts of pleasing men and attaching themselves to them to the same degree of perfection as women in our days. Some among them exhibited strong passions, but the finer sex in general did not have that inexpressible charm that freedom gives to them in the two first Nations of the universe.

However, on another occasion, that unfortunate wife consents to hateful things instead of losing all her rights:

> *Deprensum in puero tetricis me vocibus, uxor,*
> *corripis et c[ulum] te quoque habere refers.*
> *Dixit idem quotiens lascivo Juno Tonanti!...*
> *Tu Megaran credis non habuisse natis?*
> *Torquebat Phoebum Daphne fugitiva: sed illas*
> *Oebalius flammas jussit abire puer.*
> *Briseis multum quamvis aversa jaceret,*
> *Aeacidae propior levis amicus erat.*
> *Parce tuis igitur dare mascula nomina rebus*
> *teque puta cunnos, uxor, habere duos.*

– Idem. Epigrams, 44 [sic].

And there we have the Romans! One must admit however that those are not the Romans of the time of Cincinnatus, Regulus, the Fabii, or the first Cato, but just about. Long before Martial, the *Divine Augustus* had written some verse, unlike anyone else almost.

Martial, Montaigne, and M. de Voltaire have commented on that verse.

Antony[96] wrote to that same Augustus, to whom Horace said: NULLIS POLLUITUR CASTA DOMUS STUPRIS; AND, RES ITALAS ARMIS TUTERIS, MORIBUS ORNES: *Quid te mutavit? quod Reginam ineo? Uxor mea est. Nunc cœpi, aut abhine annos novem? Tu deinde solam Drusillam inis? Ita valeas uti tu hanc Epistolam cum leges, non inieris Tertullam, aut Terentillam, aut Rufillam, aut Salviam Titisceniam, aut omnes. Anne refert ubi and in quam arrigas?*

– Suetonius, Vide *Augustus*, ch. 69.

I have presented the Epigrams by the poet Martial, and some other passages, in such a way so as not to frighten my Readers. I would have abstained completely if it had not seemed necessary to me, consoling even for our century, to prove to its detractors, that it is as superior to Antiquity in the purity of its mores as in its lights. All our advantages over the Ancients are due to women. Those predilections that are frivolous in appearance, those so very seductive and diverse fashions, by augmenting their charms, bind men, preserve them from those coarse distractions against which Religion is too feeble, and which Phi-

---

[96]Antony: Mark Antony.

losophy has never helped them to avoid.

Note I

"We were approaching the Capital," said the same young man, very tired, and more bored still, "from our sojourn in a coach renowned for its slowness, when we were flagged down by two young, rather pretty persons: the first appeared to have been about twenty-four years old, and the second ten years younger. This last one had a very vivacious, bold attitude, in a word, so *grown up*, that in spite of the modesty of her chaperon she inspired in me at first some mistrust. But those mild suspicions were soon allayed. I chatted for some time with Mademoiselle *Lebrun* (that is how little *Angelique* referred to her mistress) and everything she told me was so sensible, that I was taken with much esteem for her. A young man, with whom I had struck up an acquaintance on the trip, was taken with the *Little One*; he found the favorable moment; he culled the rose... but it was not without thorns, as I learnt from him in what followed.

Note K[97]

The Abbey de Thélème by Rabelais, which M. D. D. R. regards as an imitation of public places of Prostitution, established formerly in different cities of the Realm, has, in my opinion, no relation with those houses. It is a rather amusing invention by that Author to recompense in a worthy manner a Monk of the 15th or 16th century, the Friar *Jean des Entômûres.*

After a victory, Gargantua rewards all his Captains: the last to be recompensed was the Monk *Jean*, who had not played the least part in his good success. The Prince offered him many rich Abbeys; but the friar refused, for this reason that, *as a Monk, he wanted to have neither responsibility nor government; "for, how," he said, "could I govern others, when I don't know how to govern myself."* He asked, in consideration of the service he had rendered, and those he proposed to render subsequently, that he be allowed to found a house, to which he would give a rule as he thought fit. His request having been accepted by Gargantua, the latter proposed to Friar *Jean* a beautiful stretch of land on the banks of the Loire, named *Thélème,* in order to build an Abbey there, where all that would be practiced would be the exact opposite of what is observed in other Convents.

That house will not be surrounded by walls, because Monasteries are walled; *"and not without reason,"* said the Monk, *"where with a wall before*

---

[97]Note: The original does not have a Note J. It goes from Note I to Note K.

and behind, there is great MURMUR,[98] *envy, and conspiration."* Women are not supposed to enter the monasteries of men, and it is customary in some monasteries to wash the places where they have set foot, whether they were clean or no; here, on the contrary, one will wash the places where both monks or nuns have walked. There will be no clock, because each monk will follow no other rule than his predilection or his will in the things he wants to do; not having wasted his time any more, in fact, than in monasteries where they count the hours; it is the greatest revery in the world to govern oneself by the sound of a clock, not following good sense or reason. Similarly, one ordinarily puts into Cloisters, disturbed or worthless subjects; at *Thélème* one will accept only young, alert folk, and young women will have all the perfections that make them desirable. In ordinary houses, there are only men or women; here men and women will always be together. One is engaged for one life in other Orders; here, one will be able to leave as soon as one grows tired of it.

The vows of chastity, poverty, and obedience are changed there, very nearly, into their opposite.

One is supposed to receive girls from ten to fifteen years old, and men from twelve to eighteen.

Rabelais speaks finally of the Abbey's revenues; he describes the situation and the sumptuous edifices. The inscription that one places over the portal contains an entire Chapter in burlesque verse. The Institutor wants that the *faith be founded* there, that

---

[98]Murmur: in French, the word for wall is "mur." Murmur is a pun.

error be painstakingly *banished*. After having spoken of baths, gardens, falconry, he comes to habits: nothing equals them in magnificence; one will have a habit for every season, and one will see gleaming there, *silver, gold, pearls, carbuncles, diamonds, rubies*, &c. In winter, one will dress in the French style; in spring, in the Spanish; in summer, in the Turkish; except Festivals and Sundays, wherein one will dress in the French style... Women will be in charge of the colors that men should wear. There will be a large central area next to the house, where Laborers will be lodged, who will make all sorts of beautiful objects. Employment during the day is organized by these words: DO WHAT YOU WANT: well-born persons, insofar as they are free, have in themselves a *goad* that drives them to perform virtuous acts instead of forbiddance which gives to crime the charms it would not otherwise have had; they all did, by emulation, the good they had seen done to a single person, for they could not do otherwise. Rabelais ends with this:

> *Tant noblement estoient apprins, qu'il*
> *n'estoit entr'eux celui ne celle, qui ne*
> *sçust lire, escrire, chanter, jouer d'in-*
> *struments harmonieux, parler de cinq*
> *à six langaiges, et en iceulx composer*
> *tant en carme,*[99] *qu'en oraison solue.*[100]
> *Jamais ne furent veus chevaliers tant*
> *preulx, tant galans, tant dextres*[101] *à*

---

[99]Original scholium: that is to say, in verse.

[100]Original scholium: in prose.

[101]Original scholium: adroit.

*pied & à cheval, plus vers, mieulx re-
muans, mieulx manians tous bastons
qui là estoient. Jamais ne furent veues
dames tant propres, tant mignonnes,
moins fascheuses, plus doctes[102] à la
main, à l'aiguille, à tout acte
muliebre,[103] honneste & libre,[104] que là
estoient. Par ceste raison, quand le
temps venu estoit, qu'aulcun d'icelle
Abbaye, ou à la requeste de ses parents, ou pour aultres causes voulust
issir[105] hors, auecque soy il emmenoit
vne des dames, celle laquelle l'auroit
prins pour son deuot, et estoient en-
semble mariez. Et si bien auoient ves-
cu à Theleme en déuotion & amitié:
encores mieulx la continuoient-ils en
mariage: autant s'entreaimoient-ils à
la fin de leurs jours, comme le premier
de leurs nopces.*

That resembles more the tradition of *Courtly Ro-
mance* than a Place of Debauchery. One knows that
cynical painters counted for nothing in Rabelais'
time, and that honest fellows even did not find difficulty making fun of the Works of that unrestrained
Author; Cardinal de Richelieu, it is said, received a

---

[102]Original scholium: able.

[103]Original scholium: female

[104]Original scholium: noble.

[105]Original scholium: to issue or exit.

Scholar very poorly because he confessed that he had not read them: thus it is nowise with restraint that Rabelais ends his description so modestly; but, rather, that he expressed himself just as he wished to.

One could add to that ideal Plan of Rabelais', the more verisimilitudinous Establishment of the *Virtuous Family's* Pretty-girls.

Note L[106]

Profane prostitutes, and for whom Religion was no longer the motive, have formed among all peoples a class apart. They are almost always assigned a separate location where they can practice their infamous commerce with less scandal. Public women have for a long time now attracted, even in France, the attention of the Government: there was always a certain number of them in the cities, bringing up the rear of the court, or the army, under the name of *Courtesans*, or *Ribalds*.

Letters that Charles VI in 1389, and Charles VII in 1424, gave to establish good order in places of Prostitution are recorded by Lafaille in his *History of Toulouse*. That Author says that there were in olden times in that city, and many others, a place of debauchery that was not only tolerated, but authorized even by the Magistrates, who drew an annual revenue from it. In the year 1424, because one often insulted the house that was called the *green Châtel*, and because the city was deprived of that revenue as a result of the disorder that young debauchees occasioned there, the Capitouls addressed themselves to the King

---

[106]Original scholium: In ancient Rome, one saw in places of debauchery the name of each Courtesan on her door;   whence it comes that Juvenal, speaking of Messalina, who borrowed that habit from the famous Lysisca, offered humorously, *Titulum mentita Lysiscæ... Also written on the sign was the name of the Courtesan, and the price she asked. One sees in the history of Apollonius of Tyre the form of one of those titles, which was pleasant enough*: Quicumque Tarsiam defloraverit mediam libram dabit postea populo patebit ad singulos solidos.

Charles VII, to place that house under his protection; which the King granted. The Capitouls' request would appear extraordinary today: they represented to the king, *that certain people of bad lifestyle undertook to go and break the glass panes of that house; without any fear of God.* Non verentes Deum.

In the Public Behavior Act of Narbonne, it is said that *the Consul and its inhabitants had Administration of all the affairs of police, and the right to have, in the jurisdiction of the Viscount, A RED LIGHT DISTRICT; in other words, a public place of Prostitution.*

Jeanne I, Queen of Naples, and Countess of Provence, in the *Statute of the Public Place of Debauchery* in Avignon, gives the capacity of Abbess to the Superior of Prostituted girls of that city.

I will give a report of that Rule in its entirety.

Ancient Statutes of the Public Place of Debauchery in Avignon.

1. In the year one thousand three hundred forty-seven, and in the eighth month of August, our good Queen JEANNE has permitted a Public Place of Debauchery in Avignon; and she forbids any women of debauchery to be found trafficking in the city, ordering that they be

enclosed in the Place destined for that [purpose], and so as to be recognized they should wear a red aiguillette on their left shoulder.

2. Item. If some girl who has already made a mistake wants to continue to prostitute herself, the Key-Bearer, or Captain of Sergeants, having taken her by the arm, will lead her through the city, to the sound of a drum, with the red aiguillette on her shoulder; and he will place her in the house with the others; prohibiting her to be found outside in the city, on pain of whipping on the first offense, and whipping in public and banishment if she persists.

3. Our good Queen commands that the house of debauchery be established on *Pont-troué* street, near the Convent des Augustins, as far as Porte Pieré (de PIERRE); and that on the same side there be a door through which everyone may enter, but which will remain locked, to prevent any man from going to see the women without permission of the Abbess or female Bailiff who will be elected by the Consuls every year. The female Bailiff will keep the key and will warn young people not to cause any trouble and to give no bad treatment nor fear to *women of joy*; otherwise, if there is the least complaint, they will be escorted to prison by the Sergeants.

4. The Queen wants that every Saturday the female Bailiff, and a Surgeon appointed by the Consuls, should visit each Courtesan; and if any one of them should be found who has

contracted the disease that has its origin in bawdiness, that she be separated from the others, to remain apart, so that she may not exit and spread the disease, and that one might avoid the illness that youth could pick up.

5. Item. If any of the girls should become pregnant, the female Bailiff will ensure that nothing bad happens to the child, and she will warn the Consuls, so that they might do what is necessary for the child.

6. Item. The female Bailiff will absolutely forbid any man from entering the house on Good Friday, and Holy Saturday, and the blessed day of Easter, and that, on pain of being broken, and being whipped.

7. Item. The Queen forbids women of joy from having any dispute of jealousy amongst themselves, and from stealing anything from each other, as well as fighting. She orders, on the contrary, that they live together like sisters: and if any dispute should arise between them, the female Bailiff shall settle it;

8. Item. That if someone has stolen, the female Bailiff will seek to address the theft amicably out of court; and if the girl who is culpable refuses to return what was stolen, that she be whipped in a room by a Sergeant; but if she is a repeat offender, that she be whipped by the town executioner.

9. Item. That the female Bailiff will not permit

any Jew to enter into the house; and if it should happen that a Jew, by being introduced secretly or by finesse, had had an affair with one of the Courtesans, he would be put into prison, to then be whipped on every street corner in town.

The inhabitants of Beaucaire in Languedoc had established a race where the Prostitutes of the place, and those who wanted to come to the fair of the Madeleine, ran in public the day before that famous fair, and the woman who ran best and attained the first goal given, received for a prize, a packet of aiguillettes: it is from this custom that that proverbial expression came that *a woman runs the aiguillette* meaning that she prostituted her body to everyone. It is also the custom in Italy to make Prostitutes run, and to propose a prize for the winner: we read that the famous *Castruccio de' Castracani*, General of the people of Lucca, after the battle of *Seravalle*, which he won for the Florentines, threw stunning feasts before the eyes of his enemies; and to add insult to injury he made the women prostitutes play, completely naked, at *palio* in such fashion that the vanquished could see them from atop their walls. (*That* palio *was a piece of brocade or velour, and made of other precious stuff that was won in the race.*)

Public women accompanied the troops. Brantôme says that at the rear of the Duke d'Albe's army, which Philippe II sent into Flanders against the rebels, who were reunited under the name of GUEUX, *there were four hundred Courtesans on horseback, beautiful and brave like princesses, and eight hun-*

dred on foot, well-dressed as well. La Motte-Messemé speaks of the Courtesans who brought up the rear of that army, with more detail than Brantôme. What he says is all the more curious when he reports on that together with the disposition of the many proposed Articles of Rule, which desire decency even in debauchery, and leaves out what is most contrary to nature, by giving freedom of choice as much to the public woman as to the man who chooses her. I will quote these verses, – although they can be found already in the Compilation, as learned as it is agreeable, by M. D. D. R., – so that one is not obliged to go looking for them elsewhere.

> *… Deux gaillardes Cornettes*
> *De bien trois cens chevaux à tout le moins*
>   *[complettes,*
> *Sous lesquelles marchaient des femmes de plaisir,*
> *Pour servir le premier qui en avoit desir,*
> *Pourvu, cela s'entend, qu'il leur fût agréable.*
> J'en trouvai la façon si fort émerveillable,
> Que pour les voir passer j'arrêtai longuement,
> Considérant leur port, leur grace & vétement,
> *Enrichi de couleur, sous mainte orfefvrerie.*
> J'en remarquai bien-là quelqu'une assez jolie...
> Mais plus que la blancheur le brun les
>   *[acompagne.*
> Leurs montures n'étoient de bestes de Bretagne,
> L'une avoir un cheval, & l'autre lentement
> Alloit sur un mulet, ou sur une jument:
> Les harnois néantmoins de la houtre traînante
> Sous leurs pieds, paroissoient de velours,
>   *[reluisante*

De cinq ou six clinquans cousus tout-à-l'entour,
Il les entretenoit qui vouloit tout le jour,
Mais avec un respect plein de cérémonie;
Le Barisel-major[107] leur ternit compagnie.
Or ces Dames avoient tous les soirs leur quartier
Du Mareschal-de-camp, par les mains du
                                                    [Fourrier:
Et n'eust-on pas osé leur faire insolence,
Toutefois le Duc[108] las de telle manigance.
Leur donna ce sujet de prendre meilleur parti :
Pour les malcontenter , moi-même l'entendi
Crier publiquement de mes propres oreilles,
Et Dieu sait si cela leur déplut à merveilles!
C'est qu'entre elles ne sust pas une qui osast
Refuser desormais Soldat qui la priast
De lui prester sa chambre à cinq sols par nuitée
Tâchant par ce moyen les chasser de l'Armée,
Qui lui seroit aisé, à ce que l'on disoit.
Et en avint ainsi: car telle se prisoit
Autant qu'autrefois fit cette Corinthienne...
D'en avoir fait ainsi le Duc fut estimé
D'aucuns tant seulement, des autres estant
                                                    [blasmé:
Et ceux qui admiroient en cela sa prudence,
Alléguoient que c'estoit faire une grande offense
Et desplaisante a Dieu , d'avoir incessamment
Quant & soi un tel train, de vice allechement,
Apportant à la fin, par un si grand scandale,
Des gens les mieux vivans la ruine totale,
Chascun en devisoit sélon sa passion;

---

[107]Original scholium: Prevost, or General Commander.

[108]Original scholium: d'Albe.

Car ceux-là qui tenoient contraire opinion
Ne voulant confesser bonne cette Ordonnance ,
Disoient que *le Soldat se donnerait licence*
De forcer desormais par où il passeroit
Celle qu'à son desir resister s'effayeroit,
Puisqu'il avait perdu son plaisir ordinaire,
A lui permis longtems comme MAL NÉCESSAIRE...
Mais pour ce qu'on en dit, le Duc ne retrancha
Son Edit nullement.

– *Honest Leisures* by La Motte-Messemé,
Book I, at the end.

One can only disapprove of the Duke d'Albe's expedient: the abuse that existed was incomparably less grand than what he occasioned; but what could one expect from a man who sullied his Government in the Low Lands almost every day by bloody executions? Military prostitution was debased, and became only more dangerous.

Pantagruel's prisoner in Rabelais, after the hyperbolic enumeration of his enemy forces, adds this: one hundred fifty thousand P*** (just for me, said Panurge) of which some were Amazons, others Lyonnaises, Angevines, Poitevines, Normands, Germans, from every Country, and speaking every Language.

Jean de Troyes, author of *The Scandalous Chronicle,* said that on August 14, 1465, two hundred mounted Archers arrived in Paris, following whom were eight *Ribalds*, and a *Black Monk* their *Confessor*. A pleasant equipage, and a fine office that – for the Confessor of those *Ribalds*!

Note L (bis)

The Legislator of a city in Italy (*Sybaris*), famous for its softness, forbid anyone to appear in that city bearing arms, under any pretext, that custom serving only to degenerate into bloody quarrels on the slightest dispute between the Bourgeois. *Charondas* (the name of the Legislator) sealed the law with his blood. For one day, as he was returning from the countryside, where he had found it necessary to bear arms because it was infested with brigands, he heard a great deal of noise in the city square; he thought that it was a popular uprising; he betook himself there, without noticing that he was carrying his sword. When he arrived, he realized he had made a mistake and that the assembly was peaceful. He was going to retire when someone who hated him pointed out that he had violated the law that he himself had established. "You are right," he responded to that man tranquilly; "You will see just how much I believe it is necessary," and drawing that fatal arm, he plunged it into his own chest. The Legislator thought his law was so important that he did not believe he should pardon himself for having violated it for inattention. I sense in advance that someone is going to tell me that the example of a Sybarite is not of suitable authority for us. But the Citizens of *Sparta*, those of *Athens*, and also *Rome*, will not appear to be effeminate. The greatest Warriors of all men, the most Enlightened and Victorious in our hemisphere, did not bear arms in their cities[109] and in peacetime:

---

[109]Original scholium: They had however their poignards, but the custom wasn't widespread in Rome, except during the time of the *Proscriptions*.

Cedant arma togæ.[110] says Horace. The *Barbarians* of the North, the *Huns*, the *Goths*, the *Visigoths*, the *Franks*, the *Vandals*, the *Burgundians*, the *Normands*, the *Saracens*, when they dismembered the Roman Empire while ravaging it, knew one virtue only, that of strength: their Civil Right, it was the Right of Conquest; it was quite necessary that they disarmed our fathers, after having reduced them to servitude, and that because of them they held iron in hand, always ready to cut the throat of their slaves in the event they thought to shake off their yoke. That, then, is the origin of that galant method of carrying at one's side an assassin's weapon, often fatal to whomever it was drawn on. It is the custom of the Goths, who ennobled a little the period of the Crusades or that of Chivalry: and that Gothic custom still subsists! See how ridiculous we are! Ridiculous!... and barbarous: for the bearing of arms occasions, in the Realm, the *unexpected* death of a large number of private individuals from each of the estates, and by consequence the unhappiness of many families; it occasions also the loss of the best Soldiers: in such a way that someone is not afraid to put forward that all those losses could really be shown to add up to two hundred men a year; but if it were only fifty? Does the conservation of [one hundred] fifty individuals not merit then that one suppress *effectively* and *generally* a worthless practice?

---

[110]Cedant arma togæ: arms ceding to togas.

Note M

It is certain that adornment gives women half their value. Whatever can embellish them is undertaken for them; it is their fortune; one will never be right to say that they go too far in that direction: their natural or factitious graces increase our happiness, and the sum total of our pleasures. Remove the greater part of their coiffure, their gathering corset, their pretty slipper, and what is left?... No, the honest Citizen is not at all inimical to that sort of luxury, which has no other end than to make the finer sex more enchanting, more suitable to bring to our hearts that sweet joy, legitimate voluptuousness, which is born of tender interest, a sentiment as delicious as it is inexpressible.

That a small Republic, as a Sage said, should enact *Sumptuary Laws*; that it should prevent its Citizens from taking advantage of too costly foreign stuffs, or that it should be opposed to the establishment of Manufactories that take its subjects away from the more useful labors that ought to occupy them; is reasonable. But a great Monarchy, where fortunes are necessarily of enormous inequalities, has need of luxury: France does not have the best soil in all the universe; but it is the most beautiful country in the world; and what procures it that advantage is its luxury, which makes the goods of the rich flow back into the hands of the Artist and the Artisan. All that needs to be avoided is that the luxury of cities does not tend to a depopulation of the countryside. For that then would sap the entire edifice at its foundation; but if a just proportion reigns, all goes well. There is moreover a thousand things of exquisite taste that cost much less than the labor, time, and money that went into that dreary, embarrassing, and sumptuous magnificence of our Ancestors. Man, doubtless, is the first and most handsome of the animals; but without adornment man, I repeat, would differ, my faith, much less in outward appearance than the ugliest among them. That is too well known to spend much time talking about. I consider then anything that adds to the attractiveness of the human species as something to be praised, and that it must be encouraged. When I meet an ugly man or woman, who have put much effort into their appearance, to hide the unjust caprices of nature, or the ravages of the years, I feel sincerely obliged to them: I find that they have done well to hide under a beautiful mask a face that would have saddened me. I shudder with pleasure and ravishment when I see that charming sex, on whom our pleasures and our happiness depend, join to the flowers of youth an adornment of good taste, which doubles the effect. One must be of bad humor to begrudge humankind so innocent an amusement. One knows by experience that man is to be pitied at every age: a cry of pain indicates that he is born: weakness, innumerable dangers accompany his youth: as soon as he's left home, dark pedagogues, or other tyrants, torment him like the furies until he's twenty years old: at that dangerous age, the passions dig a thousand precipices under his feet, uncertain still, and poorly assured; if he escapes, when his virtue begins to shine, envy begins to denigrate him, to pursue him to his old age: he ends then, like he began, by causing pity. Eh! deign, unjust censures, to leave him his playthings and his dolls, as long as they amuse him; there are still plenty of moments for him to feel he is unhappy!

Note N

An honest man from Province had a daughter whose pretty face and happy dispositions made him hope for consolation in his old age. His friends, in the Capital, made him understand that the young Demoiselle would receive an education much more suitable and advantageous to her in a pensione they knew of, that they would answer for. That father, whose sole concern was seeking advantages for his only daughter, entrusted her to them. Did the darling *Lucile* enter the pensione? The house was well run: the young people were always under the supervision of a Governess as good as she was enlightened and prudent: nobody left the house except with their parents, or someone sent on their behalf, and known. Who would not have thought that the young Lucile was in a safe place? Her *devotion*, a misunderstood piety, ruined her. A highly esteemed Priest was the Spiritual Director of the house. He was a man of about forty years old; with a friendly face and rather handsome. His behavior until then had been irreproachable, or, at least, none of his disorderly behavior had gotten out. The young girl had a cute face, and above all her eyes, which men who want to keep their reason should never look into. Twenty years of experience had not made the unworthy Minister of Altars any wiser: to see Lucile, to desire her, to hatch a plot to triumph over her innocence, and employee all means available, that was the result of his first meeting with her, which one calls *confession*. He took advantage then of the confidences of a young girl who opened her heart to him, and of the esteem that the entire house where she stayed had for him. Nothing was easier unfortunately; for having taken possession of her mind (and perhaps of her heart in the Tribunal) he asked whether she might be allowed to come visit him two times a week. As the house abutted the Church, Lucile went there alone; he had the skill to engage her to come to him and receive advice of the widest variety. But he made her to understand that those visits should be kept secret, so as not to make her companions jealous. Overwhelmed with preference, the young person was swimming in joy. She was only sixteen years old: more innocent at that age than a twelve-year-old girl from the Capital, she was for a long time the victim of guilty liberties before understanding a thing. Finally, emboldened by his success, the despicable Priest dishonored her. Lucile did not understand at first what ought to follow from the attempt by her abominable seducer.[111] But when the event instructed her, what despair! she wanted to kill herself; she was the victim, not the accomplice, of the monster; she disclosed without further ado all his turpitude. The two friends of her father, who happened to be in *Paris*, and whom Lucile, in her first moments of despair, informed, resolved to stab the wicked man; their plans were found out, and they were prevented from avenging an abominable crime by an unjust act, insofar as it was forbidden by the Law. The unfortunate young woman, after having deplored her unhappiness, in the most heartrending manner, went to close herself up in a re-

---

[111]A similar story, based on a true story, is told in the first part of *Thérèse Philosophe*, by the Marquis d'Argens, a contemporary of Restif de la Bretonne. See *Theresa the Philosopher and the Carmelite Extern Nun*, Sunny Lou Publishing, 2021.

treat: her father, that old man who put all his hope in her, whose daughter's misfortune was being hidden from him, surprised by her decision to renounce the world, left Province to come and see her, to make her change her mind, and lead her back with him. He arrives, asks for her: Lucile appears before him with tearful eyes, fixed on the ground; her father embraces her.

"O, my dear child," he exclaimed, "you see me and you cry!"

Lucile had a Letter all ready for him; she gives it to the author of her days: the old man reads: he grows pale; his knees buckle under him; he falls... he had just learnt everything; it was a death sentence; several days later he was laid in the coffin. *Lucile*, informed about that fatal accident, asks to exit the convent: she wants, she says. to embrace her father one last time. She is accorded that satisfaction for her tears, for her sobs. She arrives. She rushes to the inanimate cadaver.

"O you whom I loved so tenderly, and whom I have stabbed," she cried, "my father, receive me into your bosom..."

Either she had taken a dangerous potion, or her grief alone was strong enough, she collapsed onto the body of her father; she remained there; she was left there for some time. Finally, they wanted to pull her off him; she was no longer breathing... O laws! only the guilty party is still happy!

Other Books by the Publisher

Fanchette's Pretty Little Foot
by Restif de La Bretonne

Je M'Accuse...
by Léon Bloy

My Hospitals & My Prisons
by Paul Verlaine

Salvation Through the Jews
by Léon Bloy

Words of a Demolitions Contractor
by Léon Bloy

Cellulely
by Paul Verlaine

Flowers of Bitumen
by Émile Goudeau

Songs for Her & Odes in Her Honor
by Paul Verlaine

On Huysmans' Tomb
by Léon Bloy

Ten Years a Bohemian
by Émile Goudeau

The Soul of Napoleon
by Léon Bloy

Other Books by the Publisher (cont.)

Blood of the Poor
by Léon Bloy

Theresa the Philosopher &
The Carmelite Extern Nun
by Marquis d'Argens &
Anne-Gabriel Meusnier de Querlon

A Platonic Love
by Paul Alexis

Two Novellas: Francine Cloarec's Funeral
and Benjamin Rozes
by Léon Hennique

The Revealer of the Globe: Christopher Columbus
& His Future Beatification (Part One)
by Léon Bloy

Joan of Arc and Germany
by Léon Bloy

Héloïse Pajadou's Calvary
by Lucien Descaves

An Immodest Proposal
by Dr. Helmut Schleppend